The Sciatica So[...]

BANISH YOUR PAIN

AND RECLAIM YOUR LIFE

By Chet Cunningham

Foreword by: Dr. Mary Ann Castor D.C., R.N.

Agora Health Books
Baltimore, Maryland

Chet Cunningham
The Sciatica Solution: Banish Your Pain and Reclaim Your Life

Published by Agora Health Books

Alice Wessendorf, Managing Editor

Copyright 2006 by Agora Health Books
Copyright 2005/2003/2002/1997 by United Research Publishers
Library of Congress Control Number 97-60209

Previously published under the title "The Sciatica Handbook"

ISBN 1-891434-34-9
Printed and bound in the United States of America

Cover and book design by Gerrit Wessendorf

Agora Health Books
819 N. Charles Street
Baltimore, Maryland 21201
www.agorahealthbooks.com

The Sciatica Solution:
Banish Your Pain and Reclaim Your Life

By Chet Cunningham

Foreword by: Dr. Mary Ann Castor D.C., R.N.

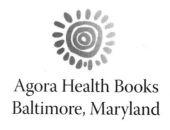

Agora Health Books
Baltimore, Maryland

DISCLAIMER

All material in this publication is provided for information only and may not be construed as medical advice or instruction. No action should be taken based solely on the contents of this publication; instead, readers should consult appropriate health professionals on any matter relating to their health and well-being.

The information and opinions provided in this book are believed to be accurate and sound, based on the best judgment available to the authors, but readers who fail to consult with appropriate health authorities assume the risk of any injuries. The publisher is not responsible for errors or omissions.

THE INFORMATION PRESENTED HERE HAS NOT BEEN EVALUATED BY THE U.S. FOOD AND DRUG ADMINISTRATION. THIS PRODUCT IS NOT INTENDED TO DIAGNOSE, TREAT, CURE, OR PREVENT ANY DISEASE.

TABLE OF CONTENTS

Foreword xi

Introduction xiii

Chapter One: What is Sciatica?   **1**

The Intervertebral Disc 2
   Why Do Discs Bulge and Rupture? 2
   The Dry Disc Dilemma 4
   The Poor Posture Connection 5
More Causes of Sciatica Pain 6
   Arthritis 6
   Ankylosing Spondylitis 7
   Spondylolisthesis 7
   Spinal Stenosis 7
   Muscle Spasms 8
   Menstrual Sciatic Pain 8
Diagnosing It 9
   Tests 9
   Other Tests 10

Chapter Two: What is Your Spine?   **13**

The Vertebrae 13
Intervertebral Discs 15
The Spinal Nerves 16

Chapter Three: Treating Sciatica the Traditional Way   **19**

Pain Pills 19
Muscle Relaxants 20

Chronic Opioid Therapy 21

Bed Rest 22

Physiotherapy 23

    Corsets / Braces 23

    Traction 24

    TENS 24

    Trigger Point Injections 25

    Ultrasound 25

    Hot and Cold Packs 25

Chapter Four: Treating Sciatica with Non-traditional Methods   27

The Mind Body Connection 28

    The Placebo Effect 28

Therapeutic Massage 29

    Chinese Massage 30

The Relaxation Response Technique 31

Biofeedback 32

Hydrotherapy 32

    Hot and Cold Compresses 33

Acupuncture 33

Acupressure 36

Reflexology 38

    Reflexology for Sciatica 39

Chiropractic 40

    Manipulation 41

    The Role of the Medical Doctor 42

    So Will Manipulation Help Your Sciatica? 43

Yoga 44

Hypnosis 46

Homeopathy 48
Osteopathy 50
   Osteopathy and Sciatica. 51
Orthopaedic Physicians 52
Supplements and Sciatica 53
   Vitamins and Minerals. 53
   Valerian Root 54
   Devil's Claw 54
   Chamomile 55
   Bromelain 55
Diet and Sciatica. 55
   Intestinal Gas and Digestive Problems 55
   Eat Your Fruits and Vegetables 56
   Bad-Back Juice Fast 56

Chapter Five: Treating Sciatica with Surgery   **59**

Decompression Surgery 60
   The Microdiscotomy 60
Spinal Fusion. 61
   Fusion Surgery 61
Chymopapain Injections 62
   Chymopapain and Sciatica 62
   How Chymopapain Works 63
   The Procedure 63
   Side Effects 64

Chapter Six: Self Help Therapy   **65**

Pain Pills 66
Heat and Cold 67
Rest Your Back 68
Alternative Approaches 68

Those First Few Exercises 71

    Walking 71

    Swimming 72

    Bicycling 72

Stress Relief 73

Chapter Seven: Yes, Exercise DOES Help   77

Warm Up Before Exercising 77

Exercise During and After an Attack 78

Stretching It Out 80

    Stretch #1: Static Hamstring Stretch 80

    Stretch #2: The Pelvic Tilt 81

    Stretch #3: Standing Pelvic Tilt 82

    Stretch #4: The Low Back Stretcher 83

    Stretch #5: Low Back Half Press Up Stretch/Rest Position 83

Back Strengthening Exercises 84

    Exercise #1: The Half Sit-Up 84

    Exercise #2: Partial Leg Lift 85

    Exercise #3: Half Squat Rotation 85

    Exercise #4: The Bridge 86

    Exercise #5: Leg Lifts While Standing 86

    Exercise #6: Abdominal Leg Extensions 87

    Exercise #7: Hand And Foot Extensions 87

    Exercise #8: Side Leg Lifts 88

    Exercise #9: Leg Lift Balance 89

    Exercise #10: Side Bends 89

    Exercise #11: Spine Rotations 90

    Exercise #12: The Resting Clam 90

    Exercise #13: Leg Thruster 90

    Exercise #14: Gentle Abs Workout 91

    Exercise #15: Holding Up The Wall 91

Exercise #16: Chair Bend Down 92
Exercise #17: The Sidewinder Slide 92
Your Exercise Plan 93

Chapter Eight: Sitting, Standing, Bending Tips   95

Poor Sitting Habits. 95
Crossing Your Legs 96
Stressful Sitting. 96
Sitting In The Same Place Too Long. 96
Slumped Over Sitting. 97
Good Sitting Habits 97
Lumbar Supports 99
Poor Standing Habits. 99
The Leaning Crane Stand 100
The Slump Stand 101
Lifting and Bending. 102

Chapter Nine: Sciatica in the Workplace   105

Your Work Station 105
Your Chair 105
Your Screen Height 106
Your Screen Distance. 107
Your Keyboard Placement. 107
Workplace Lighting 108
Try a Mini-Break 108
Heavy Labor Work Situations 109

Chapter Ten: Travel, Sleep, and Chores   111

Travel Tips. 111
Packing Up, Getting Started 111

Sleeping With A Hurting Back. 113
    Pre-bed Prepping. 114
    Time for Bed. 115
Household and Yard Work 116
    Gardening. 116
    Raking Leaves. 117
    Painting. 117
    Mowing the Lawn 118
    Shoveling Snow 118
    Vacuuming 119
    Laundry 120
    Dishes 120
    Making the Bed 120
Pregnancy and Sciatica 120

Chapter Eleven: Intimacy With a Hurting Back   **123**

A Backache Kind of Lover. 124
    Position 1 125
    Position 2 125
    Position 3 125
    Position 4 126
    Position 5 126
    Position 6 126
Getting Back in the Saddle Again 127

Appendixes and Index

Appendix I: Questions About Your Sciatica 129
Appendix II: Information Sources for Back Pain 143
Appendix III: Exercise and Aerobic Charts for Your Recordkeeping . 149
Index. XX

FOREWORD

Thousands of Americans suffer from sciatica, yet information on this subject is scarce. I visited several local bookstores and could not find a single book on the subject of sciatica.

That's why this book is of vital importance—it fills a much-needed information void for the layperson. The book explains, in easy-to-understand language, the causes of sciatica, the various treatment options available and how to help prevent possible sciatica flare-ups. The book contains a detailed section on various alternative treatments for sciatica and includes comprehensive coverage of self-help measures.

While this book is highly informative, I want to stress one point: It is not a substitute for sound professional advice. Instead, it is a valuable resource that will make you a better partner with your trained health care provider.

Dr. Mary Ann Castor, D.C., R.N.

INTRODUCTION

- Sometimes it hurts so bad you want to scream.

- It's a pain down the back of one or both legs that gives you fits.

- It hurts like fire whenever you move.

- What is it and how can you get rid of it?

We're talking about sciatica pain here. The sciatica are a pair of nerves that begin in the back inside the spinal column and run down the back of both legs all the way to the ankle. When this nerve becomes injured or is pressed upon in the spine, it can send waves of pain radiating down the lower back and the side or back of the leg and into the foot.

The pain may be only part way down one leg, or both legs, or all the way to the foot. In some cases any movement at all such as standing or walking—even coughing—will create a surge of this pain.

How you can help to reduce this pain, to live with it while it lessens and how you may be able to prevent it in the future, is the purpose of this book.

Here you'll find out exactly what sciatica is, what produces the pain, how the spine works, where the sciatica pain originates, how the spine's injury or wear and tear can produce the pain, and how sciatica can be treated with everything from diet and acupuncture to medications and in the ultimate extreme, surgery.

While sciatica pain may have any one of several causes, it is most often a result of an injury to, or wear and tear of, the discs that separate your spine's vertebrae. When operating normally these discs act as shock absorbers and separators letting your spine and your back twist and turn and move without any pain. The disc itself is made up of a soft inner core and a harder, tougher outer covering. Think about a donut with a jelly filled center and you have a good idea of what a disc in your spine is like.

Sciatica pain comes when one of the discs prolapses. This is when the soft pulpy core of the disc bulges out or is pushed out through the outer covering and presses against the sciatic nerve, which runs down the spine.

This book will go into detail about how this happens and when it does what you can do yourself to help relieve the pain. We'll show the various methods of treating sciatica, some that work and some that are little more than hype and wishful thinking and "cash cows" for the proponents.

Sciatica is often the result of bad back management, poor posture and years of misuse of your back through lifting objects the wrong way, bad sitting and standing posture and even the wrong way lying down. Since the whole back affects the spine and the discs, we'll show you the proper way to take care of your back so you'll have less chance of a sciatica attack. If you do have sciatica, this book will help you learn more about the problem, and then show you what you can do to start relieving and preventing the pain.

Exercise is a vital part of having a healthy back. But they have to be the right kinds of exercises, designed to relieve pain and tension while building muscles and avoiding injuries. To this end there are a number of exercises detailed here that show you how to strengthen your back and stomach muscles helping you to relieve and prevent that dreaded low back pain.

Putting into practice the ideas you find here, can return you to the proverbial driver's seat. You'll be armed with the knowledge and understanding you need to tackle your sciatica problems and learn to live pain free. You'll know just what to do when you start to feel those first twinges of pain and you will learn when a visit to the doctor is in order.

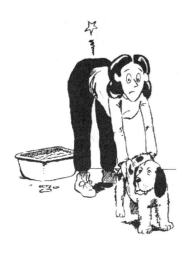

Chapter One:

What is Sciatica?

The sciatic nerve is the longest single nerve in the body. It runs through the buttocks region and down the back part of the thigh. The nerve supplies the skin of the leg, and the muscles of the back, thigh, leg, and foot.

Sciatica is a condition of the spinal column where some object, often a herniated spinal disc, is pressing against and compressing or irritating a lumbar spine root or the sciatic nerve root. The result is serious pain in the lower back and buttocks often radiating down one or both legs and sometimes all the way into the foot. Just how far the pain extends down the spinal column and into the legs depends on which disc and nerve roots are affected.

Sciatic pain can be light and periodic, or it can be so excruciatingly bad that you can't even move your legs or back without the pain surging up. The pain can be totally debilitating. The pain is often accompanied by tingling, weakness and numbness in the lower back or the affected leg.

In Germany sciatica is known as hexenschuss, which translates as witches brew. This aptly named witches pain is one that can immobilize even the toughest individuals.

Sciatica has been recorded in history down through the ages. Hippocrates, the

Greek physician, in the fifth century B.C. reported that the Scythians suffered from a lot of sciatica pain, which he attributed to their frequent horseback riding.

Roman Pliny the Elder noted five hundred years later that he had found a cure for sciatica pain. The cure, known as hiberis, was made from earthworm washings.

Sciatica even found its way into one of Shakespeare's plays in the seventeenth century. In Shakespeare's "Timon of Athens" Timon hurled the curse "Thou cold sciatica, cripple our senators."

Over the years doctors laid the cause of sciatica to a great many reasons, all which proved to be wrong until in the 1930's when two doctors discovered that sciatica was most often caused by the herniation of one or more discs in the spine.

The Intervertebral Disc

Between the vertebrae in your spine are twenty-three discs that serve as cushions to let your spine do the work it must do. Each disc acts as a joint allowing the vertebrae to move slightly as well as acting as a ligament to hold the vertebrae together. These discs are made up of a wet, spongy inner core and a stiff, sturdier outer shell that keeps the disc intact.

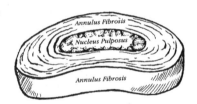

Figure 1:
Cross section view of an intervertebral disc.

Why Do Discs Bulge and Rupture?

After a person is twenty years old, these discs begin to wear in relation to the amount of pressure and movement the spine is subjected to. Many people have sciatic pain in the late twenties. It becomes more prevalent in people from thirty to fifty years of age. The age of thirty-eight is average for patients having lumbar disc surgery.

While age often is a factor, that isn't the cause of sciatica. There are a complex group of other factors that have a bearing. These include work that requires repetitive lifting, constant exposure to vibrations like long rides on a motorcycle or driving a car or truck for long periods of time. Dr. John Frymoyer in an article in The New England Journal of Medicine said that there might also be a correlation between sci-atica pain and job dissatisfaction and depression. One study even showed that ciga-rette smoking could be a risk factor leading to sciatica in some people.

Not all of the discs are prone to herniate. The two areas that are most often affected are the lumbar region, which includes the lower most vertebrae, and those high in the neck region of the spine. The lower ones are those that also bear the most weight. Both regions are subject to the greatest stress because they are mobile areas of the spine that are next to stiffer sections.

If the disc that herniates is in the neck region, it will pro-duce pain in the neck and radi-ating out into the arms some-times and all the way into the hands, resulting in numbness and muscle weakness. If the protrusion from a bulging or herniated disc touches the col-lection of nerve roots at the base of the spine called the cauda equina, the patient may

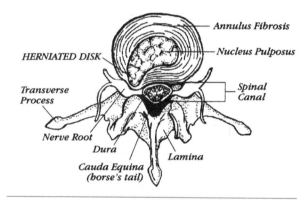

Figure 2:
Cross section of a herniated disc.

have trouble urinating or defecating. These are the nerves that control the bowels and bladder. Most sciatica problems deal with pain in the buttocks and down the legs to the feet.

When a disc herniates it is almost always the final phase of a long process of wear and tear on the disc caused by work habits, or lifting or straining. The final "blow out" of the disc might come from some innocent movement such as picking up a newspaper or bending over to sit down. In fact since the discs are designed to cushion compressive movements, but are generally weak to any twisting or rota-tional type of pressure, you are much more likely to cause a rupture of a disc with this type of injury than from a fall for example.

The Dry Disc Dilemma

When the body functions properly, the vertebral discs absorb and lose a certain amount of water and nutrients from the bloodstream. After a person is thirty years old, this balanced operation goes a little out of whack, and the discs begin to lose a little more water than they absorb. So the disc begins to dry out. This causes the width of the disc to shrink. Over the next thirty to forty years, each disc may lose up to one eighth of an inch in thickness. Multiply this times twenty-three and you see why your grandmother is shorter now then she used to be by three or four inches.

The drying out has other problems as well. If the outer layer dries out quicker than the soft inner layer, it can often result in a "leak" or rupture in the outer layer. When a leak occurs the soft inner core of the disc drains through the outer layer. When this happens the protrusion can press against the sciatica nerve root. This pressure produces the pains and discomforts of sciatica.

If the outer shell isn't broken but is bulged out by the pressure of the inner layer, the same thing can happen. The bulge of the harder layer presses against the sciatic nerve and triggers the pain. This herniated disc condition is often referred to by the public as a "slipped disc" which is incorrect. There is no slippage whatsoever of the affected disc in this case. Old labels die hard, and this condition probably will be called by this name for many years yet.

This condition almost always happens in one of the lower lumbar discs. This rupture of the disc can take place and not cause any pain, as long as the material does not press against or interfere with the work of the nerve roots. Such sciatic pain happens to about ten percent of the population. Richard W. Porter, MD, professor of orthopaedics at the University of Aberdeen in Scotland, says that only about ten percent of patients with a disc protrusion actually develop any pain from them. The other ninety percent the spinal canal is usually wide enough for the nerve to escape any damage from the bulging disc.

In some cases this bit of material that oozes out of the disc can become disconnected from the rest of the core material. Doctors then say that it is "sequestered" since it is alone. It may remain in the spinal canal and cause further problems or it may remain in place and not cause any trouble.

Usually the material from the disc core remains attached and the body starts the healing process of repairing the "leak" or bulge in the outer shell.

With the bulging disc the protrusion may not press on the nerve so much that it "pinches" it and causes it to malfunction. Many times the bulging is minor and simply irritates the nerve roots, but still causes severe pain.

Most sciatica pain is in the buttocks and legs, because of the way the nerve bundles are located. Sometimes nerves are affected which extend into the back and this will produce sciatic pain in the back as well as the lower extremities.

Such a bulging disc might cause you pain three or four times a year, and when it shrinks down the pain then goes away. These bulges might come for a variety of reasons including sim-

LOOK OUT FOR THESE RED-FLAG WARNING SIGNS

If you fit into one of these red-flag groups you should contact a doctors. These red flags may indicate a more serious problem than simple back or sciatica pain.

- Your pain is constant and getting worse
- Your pain occurred following a violent or traumatic injury such as a car accident
- You have recently lost a significant amount of weight
- You are under 20 or over 55 when you first experience the problem
- You are feeling pain in the back of your chest
- You have ever had cancer
- Your spine appears to be out of alignment
- You are experiencing numbness or loss of power
- You are on steroids

ple motions like bending forward. This can put a strain on the lower discs and cause a problem if the rear wall of the disc is weakened.

The Poor Posture Connection

A Swedish orthopaedic surgeon, Dr. Alf Nachemson, made a study of which postures and positions put the most strain on the lumbar spine discs. He found that lying on your back is least stressful with a rating of twenty-five. Lying on your side is three times as stressful, and the act of standing produces a rating of one hundred. Standing and bending over and lifting an item are more stressful with a rating of two hundred and twenty-five. Sitting and bending to the floor to pick up an object is the most stressful with a total of two hundred and seventy-five.

Curiously, sitting down is more stressful at one hundred and forty than standing is at one hundred points.

From long experience, doctors have found that a minor bulging of a disc will usually vanish along with the pain after a good night's rest. On the other extreme, some bulging discs may take three or four months to heal and for the pain to go away. Doctors say that even the most severely herniated disc should heal after nine months. Most sciatic pain should be gone after sixty days.

More Causes of Sciatica Pain

While the ruptured or bulging disc is perhaps the most common cause of sciatica pain, it can also be triggered by infections, injuries, tumors, arthritis, ankylosing spondyltis, a condition known as spondylolisthesis, spinal stenosis and even muscle spasms. Let's check out some of these other possible causes of the pain.

Arthritis

There are three types of arthritis that affect the spine: degenerative arthritis, osteoarthritis and rheumatoid arthritis. Degenerative arthritis is by far the most common and at the same time usually the least serious. This is a normal part of the aging process. This simply means that as we get older, the more our joints wear and some of them wear out. The problem is that the cartilage that cushions and protects the joints wears away. The joints most affected include the hands and feet and the spine.

When the cartilage wears thin and the discs shrink down because of age and wear and tear, there's more chance of the sciatica nerve roots in the spinal canal being affected.

Osteoarthritis is the growing of rims or bony spurs either on or near the facet joints. Interestingly these spurs may actually help stabilize the discs or joints of the spine and may help you avoid back pain, not cause it. In people over sixty-five this condition may limit mobility and cause some stiffness of the back. However osteoarthritis is not a big factor in back pain and rarely is there any serious problem involved.

Rheumatoid arthritis can attack the spinal column, but it also is a body wide disease affecting the joints in the hands, elbows, fingers, toes and shoulders as well. If it affects the facet joints of the spine, it results in severe inflammation, swelling and painful stiffness. Rheumatoid arthritis can destroy the joint as it progresses as well as the tissue surrounding it.

Ankylosing Spondylitis

This is a severe inflammation of the spinal joints that then stiffen and cause severe pain. Ankylosing Spondylitis usually starts at the base of the spine and works its way upward. Twice as many men are affected as women and it usually starts in the late twenties. As it progresses, the vertebrae fuse and the victim hunches over until he can hardly see ahead.

Spondylolisthesis

Spondylolisthesis is the real slipped disc. For this to happen, first there must be a crack in the back of a vertebra. When this crack widens sufficiently, the front section of the vertebra can then slip forward in relation to the vertebra below it. In a mild form this problem can go unnoticed since there is little or no pain involved. A flare up of pain may come from sudden exertion. The best treatment is exercises to strengthen the area after the pain subsides.

Spinal Stenosis

Another way that sciatica pain can develop is from spinal stenosis. This means narrowing and here applies to the narrowing of the spinal canal through which the sciatica nerve passes. This problem comes with the advent of degenerative arthritis when the formation of bone spurs on the spine can change the contours of the vertebrae.

There are a wide variety of ways that this narrowing affects the sciatic nerve depending where the narrowing takes place. It can mean the tingling, numbness and the shooting pain and weakness usually associated with sciatica.

GOOD TO KNOW

As the sciatic nerve leaves the pelvis it passes near a muscle called the piriformis that lies deep within the buttocks. It is estimated that in 10% to 15% of the population the sciatic nerve actually passes through the piriformis muscle leaving this group much more susceptible to having sciatic problems. Piriformis Syndrome is responsible for at least 6% to 8% of sciatica cases.

Muscle Spasms

Muscle spasms resulting from an injury or just a fall can irritate the sciatic nerve. Some experts say, for example, that an inflamed piriformis muscle in the buttocks can press against the sciatic nerve and cause the pain. This muscle is the one that lets you lift your leg sideways. The piriformis can become inflamed from an injury or over-exertion.

Menstrual Sciatic Pain

On some rare instances other causes can trigger sciatica pain. A case in point. A woman in Tokyo went to her doctor about sciatica pains coinciding with her menstrual cycle. She said she had severe right-side sciatica that began a day before her menstruation began, peaked two days into the cycle and then gradually ebbed away over the next fourteen days. After that she was pain free until two days before the next cycle.

The doctor's X-rays showed nothing. Her blood cell count, blood chemistry and erythrocyte sedimentation rate were all normal.

A CT scan of her lumbar spine showed a small disc herniation between the L5 and S1 vertebral levels. The doctor discounted this as the source of the pain.

Further CT scanning showed a large mass in the pelvic cavity. More testing showed it to be an endometrioma. The doctor shrank the endometrial cyst and the woman's sciatic symptoms vanished.

This cause of sciatica pain is rare, but if all else fails it could be an area to investigate.

Diagnosing It

When you have a serious back pain and go to your doctor, he will start by taking a history of your back problem. Doctors tell us that it is difficult to diagnose a bulging disc quickly. He will start by asking you several questions. He'll ask if you've had any work where you had to do a lot of lifting or if you've had any recent falls or injury to your back or legs. Most doctors agree that pinpointing the cause of back pains is difficult.

If the sudden pain is "electric" and results in a burning sensation and sometimes numbing and tingling, it usually is determined to be sciatica and not the milder buttocks and leg pain from a facet joint problem.

Sciatica pain usually is more severe when bending forward and when coughing or sneezing and this is another way to help diagnose it. By flexing the neck forward increased stress is placed on the spinal cord. If there is a herniated disc, such neck flexing can create a sharp pain down the legs or in the buttocks, and sciatica is the diagnosis.

Tests

A physical examination should be a part of every doctor's evaluation of a person with back pain. Here are some of the tests that your doctor is likely to perform before making a diagnosis.

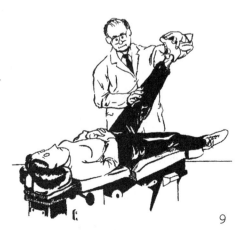

Straight Leg Lift Test. This is performed with you lying flat on your back with feet fully extended. The examiner lifts one of your legs at a time to see if you experience any pain. If there is a sciatica problem, usually pain will shoot down the affected leg when it is reaches an angle from about twenty-five to seventy-five degrees. When your leg is lifted this way it stretches the nerve roots at the spinal cord and they are put under increased tension, which causes the pain.

Related Pain Test. If pain courses down one leg when the other leg is being raised, it is another indication of sciatica with the added problem of a disc fragment. In this case a piece of the herniated disc may have broken off and is pressing against the sciatic nerve root.

The Lasegue Test. In this test your ankle and foot are pushed up toward the knee. This will put further stress on the nerve roots and if there is a problem with a disc, will cause you intense pain.

Neurological Examination of Leg. For this exam a pinwheel or other neurological tool is used to test any nerve problem in the leg, thigh or foot. Here too, reflexes at the back of the ankle and the knee will be tested and evaluated.

Motor Strength Test. The motor strength will be tested in your leg, ankle and foot in one or both legs and the results evaluated.

Lumbar Area Motion and Range Test. The range and motion of the lumbar spine area will be tested as well as the route of the sciatic nerve going down the leg for tenderness or spasms.

These tests will not only confirm or rule out a sciatic problem, but will help the examiner to figure out just which disc is affected.

Other Tests

If your doctor tries all the above tests and does not find an indication of a herniated disc, or if he wants confirmation of some of his findings he may order some additional test.

X-Ray: Taking X-rays of the lumbar region of your spine is a quick and inexpensive way to check for problems with your lower back; however, they simply can't detect a ruptured disc. That's because the regular X-ray shows bones, and bone structure; they can't show the soft tissue of which the disc is made.

What X-rays can show are other problems with your back and spine such as cancer, fractures in your spine, or arthritis damage to the vertebrae. If your pain continues, your doctor may start the testing with an X-ray just to rule out other problems.

CAT Scan: The next test your doctor may try could be a computerized tomographic scan, CT or often called a CAT scan. Again it will pinpoint the lower back and the lumbar vertebrae since this is where sciatica pain is caused.

Most specialists say that a CAT scan can find 75% of herniated discs when they are taken properly. The CAT scan is not without some distortion and some disc problems may seem to be there when there is nothing wrong. But it's the best test we have right now.

A CAT scan is done in the radiology department of a hospital or clinic. It's an outpatient procedure and no hospitalization is required. The patient wears a hospital gown and is placed on a platform that is slowly moved into a large circular device that encloses the person. The CAT scan is painless.

As the patient is slowly' drawn through the large tube, a scanner is taking millions of readings by special types of rays that result in a print out of a perfect picture of the area, in this case the spine. A computer prints out pictures of the area and a diagnosis is made.

The pictures from this machine will show the discs between the vertebrae and in about 75 percent of the cases the radiologist can determine if there is a herniated disc or not.

The scanner gives out cross sections of the spine less than a quarter of an inch thick. With the computer scanner the interior of the bones can be evaluated. The computer reconstructs the views of the scanner and comes up with the precise areas that the radiologists asks it to.

A CAT scan involves radiation and since a session might take a half hour or more, some patients wonder about being overexposed to the radiation. Actually the radiation comes in brief strobes and an entire CAT scan will typically give a patient no more radiation exposure than four or five regular X-rays.

Magnetic Resonance Imaging:
The MRI is another method of testing for a herniated disc. Using a magnetic field and radio waves signals are produced that are then converted into images of your body by a computer. Some specialists say the MRI is better at finding ruptured discs than the CAT scan. One drawback is the cost. An MRI can cost from about $600 to as much as $4,000 depending on what is tested and how long it takes.

TAME THE PAIN TIP

Never twist your body to the side when lifting or lowering an object and always bend your knees when picking up or putting down an object.

Most MRI's will find a herniated disc in 90 percent of the cases.

The MRI is painless and there is no radiation exposure to worry about. It works through the use of magnetic rays, which are harmless. Again, this is an outpatient procedure and no hospitalization is needed. There are no injections or medications and any risk factor is extremely low.

The MRI can help detect cancer, infection and fractures in the spine as well as herniated discs. Sometimes it can give a false image of a ruptured disc when it isn't there. The MRI and the CAT scan are the best diagnostic tools we have so far for the disc problem.

The Myelogram: A myelogram is a test that uses a radiopague fluid that is injected directly into the spine cavities near a suspected ruptured disc or other spinal problems. The fluid is impervious to X-rays. Now the X-rays will highlight problems with the discs that a straight X-ray could not.

The myelogram can leave a patient with a headache and dizziness but some patients experience no side effects at all. As with any invasive procedure, the myelogram carries with it a small element of risk to the patient. It is also uncomfortable for the patient.

Many doctors prefer using a CAT scan over a myelogram because it is simpler, less invasive, easier on the patient and usually just as good or better results can be obtained.

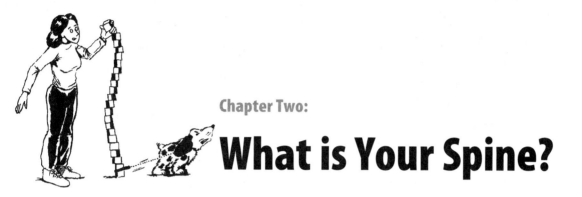

Chapter Two:

What is Your Spine?

Before we get into too much detail here about the sciatica problem and ways to handle it, let's do some basic training and take a good look at the spine—that's where this problem centers and we need to know as much about it as we can.

The spine or backbone is the major bone structure of your back. Sometimes called the vertebral column by doctors or scientists, every other part of your back and your whole rib cage is hung on this spine. The backbone houses and protects the spinal cord.

The Vertebrae

The basic building block of the back is called the vertebra. It's a relatively small bone, only a few inches wide. However, this group of twenty-three vertebrae does a tremendous job of permitting the human body to bend and twist and do all sorts of complicated maneuvers without breaking. The word itself comes from the Latin word vertere, which means to turn.

The vertebrae have been honed and sculptured and tailor made to their tasks down through millions of years of evolution into three dimensional building blocks that do at least four vital functions in your back.

Just like building blocks, the vertebrae are stacked up in order, some larger than others and each group designed for specific purposes. The stack of vertebrae forms a strong column, or backbone, that is designed to support the considerable weight of the upper body.

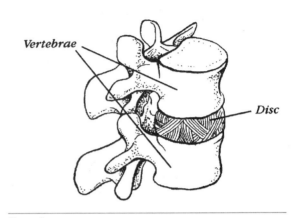

Figure 3:
Illustration of the vertebrae in the spine.

The body of the vertebra is nearly circular in shape. It has a hole through it on the backside and these holes are all aligned to form a smooth vertical hole or tunnel from top to bottom. This is called the spinal canal and it contains and protects the spinal cord through which all of the major nerves from the brain run to the rest of the body.

The vertebrae are joined together in a vertical stack by the facet joints. These fairly flat surfaces slide over each other to some extent to permit some movement. By the same factor, they also limit how far you can bend or twist your back.

Medical people divide this stack of vertebrae into three main sections. The top six vertebrae are called the cervical ones. These serve the neck and end about at the top of the shoulders.

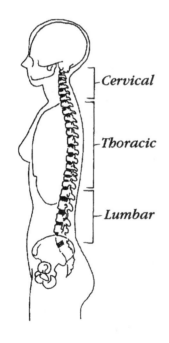

Figure 4:
The vertebrae in the spine are divided into three main stacks that add up to form the natural curvatures of the spine.

The next twelve are named the thoracic vertebrae. These go from the shoulders almost to the bottom of the rib cage. The remaining bones and discs are named the lumbar vertebrae and extend to just above the hipbones.

The lumbar vertebrae are the ones that we are the most concerned with, since this is where the majority of the problems occur that result in sciatica.

If you looked at a spinal column from the front, it would appear to be a straight vertical stack of bones with no curves to the right or left. However if you look at the same spine from the side, you'll see that it does have several curves.

Through the neck area there is the cervical curve that swings slightly backwards from the chest. Just below that in the thoracic vertebrae the curve reverses itself and now swings outward toward the chest. Just below the rib cage the lumbar curve swings the spine again toward the back. Below the hipbones the sacral curve moves the spine all the way to the tailbone in a forward curve again. These curves must be in the right places and in the right form for your spine to function normally.

Intervertebral Discs

Another important part of the spinal column we are interested in here are the discs that are situated between the bottom and tops of each vertebra and cushion and serve as shock absorbers for the spine. We already discussed discs briefly in Chapter One.

These "pillows" between the vertebrae are about a quarter of an inch in thickness, maybe more in some people and less in others, and they will also vary in width from one vertebra to the next depending where it is in the spinal column and how much pressure is on it.

These discs are what compress and expand to allow the spinal column to bend and shift with the stretching and workloads the muscles attached to it accept.

The discs will shrink in their thickness during the day when the body is pushing down on them for hours at a time. But at night they will be unpressured and will revert back to their original size. Some people are from a half to three quarters of an inch shorter after an active day, than they were when they got out of bed that morning.

Discs are composed not of bone but of a substance similar to the cartilage that forms your ears and nose. In the discs it is slightly yellowish and is called fibro-cartilage.

> ## TAME THE PAIN TIP
>
> Sitting incorrectly can lead to back pain. Avoid sitting in a twisted or leaning position in a chair. Sit upright, facing forward, and with your feet flat on the ground. If your feet do not reach the floor you should use a cushion or footstool.

The disc has two main parts, the inner core, and a pulpy and soft mass named the nucleus pulposus. The outer part of the disc is made up of parallel fibers that are harder and hold the core in place. This is called the annulus fibrosus. Think of a jelly donut with the jelly as the core and the outside of the donut holding the jelly in as the outer ring.

The discs are more than eighty percent water. This is what permits them to hold the pressure and to be elastic so they can let the spine bend on call. The disc can change shape rather drastically and then when the spine removes the pressure, the disc returns to its original shape.

The high water content lets the disc absorb blows and jolts to the upper body. That's the reason the discs are called the shock absorbers for the spine.

The Spinal Nerves

We are vitally concerned with the nerves that run through this vertical spinal canal. Those nerves are what send many men and women straight up the wall with sciatica pain.

This canal runs the entire length of the spinal column from the base of the brain downward. Inside this sheath in the canal run a sensitive bundle of hundreds of nerve cells and fibers. They form a group about as thick as a man's small finger. This group of nerves is the super highway of communications from the brain to the body.

Nerves branch off from the main stem to meet the needs of every body part. They go at regular intervals in pairs on each side of each of the vertebrae. They are called nerve roots. There are thirty-one pairs of nerve roots emanating from the spinal cord.

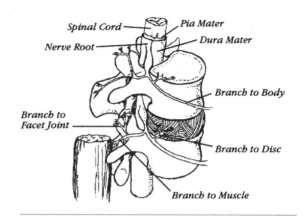

Figure 5:
The spinal nerves branch off from the main stem to service every part of the body.

Each set of nerves is designed to service a specific part of the body. They soon branch out and combine and branch again until that part of the body is completely serviced with nerve endings. For example the nerves between the fourth and fifth neck vertebrae serve the muscles that let you move your shoulders and upper arms.

The nerves exiting from between the fourth and fifth lumbar vertebrae leave the hips and go down each leg to activate the hips and knees. Those from between the fifth lumbar and the sacrum let us move our feet.

These nerves that control the legs and feet combine high up and bundle together as they work down from the hips are called the sciatic nerve. This nerve is where the trouble can come from if you suffer from sciatica pain.

So, that's the human spine, a marvelously wonderful structure that we're going to be talking about a lot during this discussion of sciatic pain and what you can do about it.

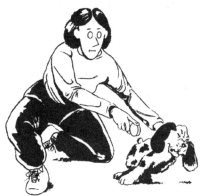

Chapter Three:

Treating Sciatica the Traditional Way

Whenever you experience severe pain the first thing you should do is check in with your doctor to rule out cancer and other serious ailments. This will give you some peace of mind that your problem is indeed sciatica, it's not fatal and there are several ways to deal with it.

First your doctor will diagnose the problem. Most likely he will do some of the tests we talked about in the previous chapter. Next most doctors will take the less invasive path suggesting you go home, take some pain pills, give your back a day or two of rest and then see how you feel. Many times this will reduce or eliminate the pain and nothing more will need to be done.

Pain Pills

When it comes to pain medications start with the simplest non-prescription forms and see if they work for you before moving on to the heavier prescription stuff. Take the lowest dosage of the mildest pill you can take that does the job for you. No pain medication, even the over-the-counter variety, should be taken without a doctor's advice for more than ten days.

The simplest is any of the common aspirins on the market. From the supermarket bottle of 500 to the fancy wrapped package of a name brand, all do about the same thing. They are anti-inflammatory analgesics that pave the road for tissue repair as well as relieving your pain.

Other over-the-counter pain relievers you are surely already familiar with are the ibuprofens like Advil and Motrin and the naproxen sodium tablets such as Aleve. All of them will help reduce pain and at the same time allow for your body to start the repair procedures, patching up your ruptured disc or reducing inflammation around the disc.

As always be sure to follow the directions on the box for dosage and length of use. The main advantage of these drugs is that they contain no opiates, there is no risk of addiction, and this is very important to those with any kind of chronic pain.

Muscle Relaxants

When you start talking about medications to relax the muscles you are moving into the realm of prescription drugs that contain narcotics. The big danger here is getting addicted to the pills so that you can't do without them.

These include drugs such as Percodan, Rbaxisal, Tylenol-2, Tylenol-3 and Tylenol-4. Tylenol-2 contains fifteen mg of codeine. The Tylenol-3 has thirty mg of codeine and the 4 has sixty mg of codeine. Codeine is easy to become addicted to yet most people don't even realize that it can be a threat.

GOOD TO KNOW

To avoid any possible medication interactions it's a good idea to keep a listing of all your medications as well as any vitamins or nutritional products you are taking in your wallet. When your doctor wants to prescribe a medication or pain reliever he will have any easy reference to check first.

A note of warning. If you use more than one doctor, such as a GP and a neurologist, be sure that you tell each what medications you are taking so they are not duplicated and so no medications are prescribed that together can cause bad side effects or even be deadly. Anytime you get a new prescription filled, tell your pharmacist what other medications you're taking and ask him if any of them should not be taken at the same time. He'll know.

The rule with any medication: use as little as you can to get the job done, and use it for as short a time as possible.

Chronic Opioid Therapy

Chronic opioid therapy is relatively rare therapy that is sometimes used in uncontrollable chronic pain cases. This is the practice of prescribing potentially very dangerous drugs such as morphine and high potency codeine that while very effective are also highly addictive. While this therapy is more often prescribed in cases like terminal cancer it is not unheard of for it to be used in chronically bad back pain cases when a doctor cannot find any other effective method for relieving the pain.

Doctors who use this therapy say there are a certain percentage of back pain patients who can undergo this therapy with no substance abuse issues and no addiction problems. They maintain that they are very careful about who they prescribe it for.

However, even if the patient doesn't develop an addiction there is still the issue of severe side effects. Side effects of this therapy include persistent constipation, insomnia, lowered sexual desire and function and even trouble thinking clearly and focusing.

Doctor's often use a mental checklist, similar to the one below, before prescribing any chronic opioid treatment:

- ☐ all other reasonable attempts at pain control have not worked
- ☐ the patient does not have any history of drug abuse
- ☐ as the prescribing doctor I will take personal responsibility for the patient and follow up with him weekly
- ☐ I have received a written informed consent prior to starting this treatment

- ☐ dosages will be on an around-the-clock basis
- ☐ if this patient does not receive partial pain relief after the first few low doses this treatment will be stopped
- ☐ I will look for any evidence of drug abuse or addiction and will immediately stop treatments if there is any sign of either

Bed Rest

Most older books and manuals on back problems tout bed rest for from two weeks up to a month as a basic treatment for many patients. Now doctors have changed that policy. Specialists currently say that one or perhaps two days of bed rest after a shattering bout with sciatica or other back problems is as much as you should do.

Too much bed rest can actually cause problems. Some regimens just ten or fifteen years ago called for six to eight weeks of bed rest. Most doctors now say that this is far too much; one to three days is more realistic.

Too much time in bed can lead to all sorts of problems including weakening of the muscles and a tendency to soften the bones. It can cause depression, stomach and bowel upsets, loss of bone and mineral tissue, blood clots in the legs, weakening of the spine's discs, cartilage and ligaments.

Bed rest doesn't mean total immobility. Rest your back, but don't worry about getting out of bed two or three

TAME THE PAIN TIP

Exercise is a great way to relieve any type of chronic pain including sciatica. Inactivity leads to muscle atrophy and a loss of strength. But movement can build strength and flexibility while causing a feel-good endorphin release. Other side benefits include better sleep, higher energy levels, and weight loss. So get moving!

times a day. Going to the bathroom is fine but get right back to bed for that day or two. Get up for meals, but don't over do it.

Physiotherapy

After your doctor has checked you, done tests to be sure there are no serious causes of your back pain such as a tumor or a cancer, and determines that there is no need for surgery, most medical doctors then pass the patient on to a physical therapist.

Physiotherapists are schooled in a variety of methods and treatments that can help you get rid of your back pain. A few of the more common methods are discussed below. However this are probably dozens of other treatments your therapist may choose to use in your treatment.

Corsets / Braces

A corset will provide support for an injured back. There are both long corsets used for pain in the mid to the lower thoracic spine area and short corsets used for low back pain. These are called lumbar or lumbosacral braces.

A medical corset is essentially a type of back brace, which often extends over the buttocks area and may be held in place by shoulder straps. Like an old-fashioned woman's corset they often lace up either down the sides or on the front or back of the brace. Two common braces are the Boston Brace and the Raney Flexion Jacket.

A brace may be prescribed in severe back pain cases, but it is advisable to limit their use, since using them for extended periods of time can allow abdominal muscles to weaken and atrophy.

These braces are designed for good abdominal compression and for a minor flexed lumbar spine. This lumbar flexing can decrease the backward bulge of a disc and relive some of the pressure on the lumbar spine's rear elements. When wearing a brace you are constantly reminded to restrict sudden movements.

Any lumbar brace you buy is going to be expensive. Just the nature of the beasts. These are not used as much today as they were in the past and you might have trouble finding them in some areas. Be sure this is what you need before you go this route.

They have some other drawbacks. Braces can irritate bony prominences in your back as well as your skin. Sometimes a back brace will cause more pain instead of lessening it.

Traction

Traction is usually used in a hospital or therapy situation where ropes pull one part of your body one way while other ropes pull it the opposite direction. Once used extensively for sciatica, several clinical studies indicate that traction does little if any good at all for sciatica and most back problems.

There are still some proponents of traction in back pain cases and under the guidance of a therapist it should do no harm. So if other methods have not worked for you and you want to give it a try go right ahead.

TENS

Transcutaneous Electrical Nerve Stimulation or TENS, as a method of relieving pain first became popular in the 1960's. In the case of severe back pain electrodes were surgically inserted into painful areas of the back and activated with low charges of electricity.

Obviously this method, requiring surgery, was invasive and soon a non-invasive method was created in the form of a TENS machine. The TENS machine is a portable battery powered machine that can be worn around the waist that has electrodes that are taped to the skin. The electric current is delivered from the battery pack on an on-demand basis by the user.

There are two basic types of TENS machines. In one the current that is used resembles a buzz, the other is more like a gentle and nudging electric shock. The electrodes are placed on the back in a number of places until the best spots are located.

Often used for chronic back pain, the TENS treatment is said to give relief from pain in about a third of the patients. Experts say that the electric current's high frequency stimulates the large sensory fibers. This lessens the patient's sensitivity to the pain as it travels along the smaller sensory fibers.

Trigger Point Injections

Sometimes pain in the back can be very specifically pin pointed. Pressing on a specific point triggers more pain for the sufferer.

Some therapists use injections of local anesthetic into such trigger points, such as cortisone or saline, to relieve pain. This method does often give quick relief, but it is not permanent. However during these periods of relief, the therapist may be able to use other methods of treatment that were not practical before.

There is no solid evidence that such injections will work for everyone, however if it works for you, be thankful. Be sure the needles are sterile and the injections are given correctly.

Ultrasound

Your physical therapist or doctor may suggest ultrasound in some situations to reduce pain and stimulate healing. Ultrasound delivers high frequency sound waves of over a million cycles per second into targeted tissue. This is the same as ultrasound used for diagnostic work, but the wattage is much lower and the heat generated is less.

The ultrasound vibrates individual cells in the body. This is thought to cut down on the pain by activating the large sensory fibers so the relatively few pain messages working along the small fibers are not as recognized—hence less pain is felt.

Ultrasound can also help break down scar tissue and at the same time activate new connective tissue. Ultrasound will also change the characteristic of the cell walls. With heightened permeability, the cell can rid itself of waste products easier and nutrients can be absorbed quicker. This means an inflamed area will see healing take place faster.

Hot and Cold Packs

Hot packs, moist or dry, should not be used on a new injury. But after the injury is moderated, hot packs can help bring new blood into the region and help stimulate healing. The heat is soothing to any injury and with the increase in blood supply and oxygen it will help decrease muscle tension. Heat can also stimulate the large sensory fibers decreasing the perception of pain.

Cold packs are often used to reduce swelling. There is little swelling in a sciatic pain situation, but the cold pack can still be helpful. It reduces the circulation to the area when used. If it is alternated with a hot pack the new infusion of blood will be greater than with the hot pack alone. If you find a hot pack is more painful than soothing, try switching to a cold pack.

Generally an ice pack should not be placed directly on the skin and should not be used for more than fifteen minutes at a time. A great idea for an instant ice pack is to grab a bag of frozen peas from your freezer and wrap them in a cloth. The peas are pliable and will mold nicely around the curves in your back and when they melt you can just toss them back into the freezer.

TAME THE PAIN TIP

To soothe pain and ease swelling and inflammation you can use a commercial cold pack or make your own homemade cold pain-reliever:

- To make an ice towel wet a towel with cold water and squeeze out the excess water until it is just damp. Fold the towel, place it in a plastic bag, and put it into the freezer for at least 15 minutes. Remove the bag, wrap in a light towel or cloth, and place it on the affected area.

- To make an ice pack. Put about 2 to 3 cups of ice into a large plastic freezer bag and add water so it just covers the ice. Squeeze the air out of the bag and seal it. Wrap the bag in a cloth and apply it to the affected area.

- To make a homemade slush pack mix about 3-cups water and 1-cup denatured alcohol in a sealable freezer bag. Close the bag and place it into the freezer until a slush forms. Wrap the bag in a cloth and apply it to the affected area.

- Try a bag of frozen peas as a cold pack. Wrap the frozen bag of peas in a cloth and apply to the affected area.

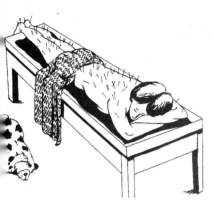

Chapter Four:

Treating Sciatica with Non-traditional Methods

There are millions of people who believe passionately in non-traditional forms of healing of mind and body. If you aren't one of them, look at these "different" forms of healing and maintaining your spine and your back with a good deal of common sense. Some of them might work for you. Some of them might trigger a placebo effect that will be tremendously worthwhile for you. Some of them may have inherent curative powers. Some of them might not work at all for you.

For a great many years, in the United States in particular, the medical community looked with extreme disfavor on any type of treatment for a known medical disease or problem or condition that did not follow the normal general medical practices. Thankfully these views are finally starting to change and attitudes are beginning to loosen. Many people are choosing to seek out naturopathic physicians these days. These medical professionals specialize in natural healing methods and are trained at accredited medical schools.

GOOD TO KNOW

For a referral to a naturopathic physician you can visit The American College for Advancement in Medicine (ACAM) at www.acam.org (or call 1-800-532-3688) or The American Association of Naturopathic Physicians at www.naturopathic.org (or call 1-866-538-2267).

You must be the final judge and jury. It all boils down to this. If it's traditional or non-traditional, if it works for you, run with it and don't do a lot of worrying about why.

The Mind Body Connection

There is little doubt that the mind can have a physical effect on the body. People can essentially "think themselves sick". Anyone who has experienced the effect stress can have on their health (and who hasn't?) can attest to the powerful connection our mind has to our physical well-being. While the mind and body relationship has not been honed to an exact science even the traditional world of medicine generally has the attitude of "If it works, if it helps heal the body and is beneficial to the patient, let it happen."

The Placebo Effect

For a great many years doctors themselves have used a technique in medical studies where one set of patients is given a new medication. The other half of the patients with the same medical condition are given sugar pills, the so-called placebo.

Medical researchers say that the placebo group of patients should not realize any benefit whatsoever from the pills. They maintain that the placebos are simply good tasting sugar pills. Much to the surprise and sometimes chagrin of researchers, there always are a percentage of the placebo patients who show improvement when taking

GOOD TO KNOW

Most people believe that placebos are made of inert substances and are designed to have no effect. However, the fact is that there is no such thing as an inert substance and even sugar, as anyone who has felt a sugar high before can attest, has an effect on the body. In addition it may surprise you to know that pharmaceutical companies actually produce their own placebo pills choosing their own ingredients and they are not required to disclose what those ingredients are. Some placebos are even designed to be "active placebos" that mimic the side effects of the tested drug so that the control groups and placebo groups will have similar experiences.

the inert sugar pills in a closely controlled, double blind, testing situation.

It has come to be known as the placebo effect, and is pushed into the realm of the psychiatrist who tells us that some people can effect "cures" and "benefits" and improvements" in their condition in a great variety of ailments, simply by believing that they are receiving medication that will generate these improvements in their condition.

Closely allied with the placebo effect is the psychosomatic situation. Psycho-somatic is simply the result of bodily symptoms that are caused by mental or emo-tional disturbances. You've heard of a psychosomatic illness—when a person starts to believe that he or she has a physical problem and they absolutely know they have it and soon they develop the physical symptoms of that disease or problem. Medical doctors can become extremely mixed up by such symptoms only to find with tests that the person actually doesn't have the disease at all.

Therapeutic Massage

While therapeutic massage is a common practice used by physical therapists in the treatment of pain and back problems it still sits just on the other side of the traditional non-traditional therapy line. There are hundreds of thousands of men and women who swear by a good massage as a way to gain relief, even if tempo-rary, from any number of back pains and aches and troubles including sciat-ica and studies in the last couple of years are beginning to back them up.

The massage therapist uses her

GOOD TO KNOW

One study, published in the April 23, 2001 issue of the ARCHIVES OF INTERNAL MEDICINE evaluated the effec-tiveness of therapeutic massage for chronic back pain. The study includ-ed 262 participants, ages 20 to 70, each of which had seen their doctor in the past six weeks for persistent back pain problems. Each was ran-domly assigned to receive therapeu-tic massage, traditional Chinese medical acupuncture, or self-care educational materials. After 10 weeks researchers found that mas-sage was superior to self-care and acupuncture. The massage group used the least medications and had the lowest costs of subsequent back care.

hands or specialized tools, to rub, knead, and stroke the affected areas. The massage is designed to eliminate stress and tension while increasing blood flow and oxygen to the area to speed healing. In addition it is thought to help eliminate acids and other waste products that have accumulated helping to relieve pain.

How else might massage help with back pain? An injury in the back can mean that some muscles go into spasm to protect the injured area. The spasm becomes a kind of splint giving that protection. Once the injured area is healed, the "splint" of spasming muscle should relax. Often this doesn't happen.

Massage can be used to help relax the muscle. However since the spasm was in place for some time, it can often return with the slightest increase in pressure or stress on the former injury. A number of massages may be needed to permanently relax that particular muscle and keep it in a natural state.

Some of the best massage therapists gladly work with, not against, medical doctors. Many will encourage their patients with back problems to exercise and improve their posture.

If it works for you, use massage.

There is a growing belief in the healing world that simply being touched by another person can have nourishing and healing benefits. The idea of touching as a method for pain relief is becoming more recognized. One massage therapist said: "An exchange of energy is involved in the touching aspect of massage. It can help a person feel less alone and more connected to the world."

Chinese Massage

Traditional Chinese Medicine (TCM) has been used for over 2,000 years to cure disease in China. Chinese Massage is often used for pain relief. This ancient therapy is based on channels or meridians that energy is thought to use to flow through the body. TCM is built on the concept of balance, Ying and Yang, and with the two essential substances, Qui and blood. In TCM it is believed to cure a disease you must cure its root.

Back pain is believed to come from an invasion of Cold and Damp, or from a result of weakness of the kidneys, neurosis, exhaustion or frequent sexual intercourse. Chinese Massage for back troubles is designed to strengthen the back and the kidneys. It also improves Qui-blood flow and expels Cold and Damp. Using pain-relief points and various manipulations the Chinese Massage practitioner works to relieve pain and to cure disease.

In a typical Chinese Massage for back pain your practitioner will often start by working with acupoints on each side of the back of the neck, squeezing them with thumb and fore finger. He then may manipulate the acupoints on the back of each shoulder half way between the neck and the outside of the shoulder. Next he may work to open channels in the back region. These acupoints are near the bottom of the back and low down and on one side.

If this type of therapy interests you, by all means get a good book on Chinese Massage and start learning more about it.

The Relaxation Response Technique

There may be a way you can reduce the pain of your sciatica or your back simply by doing nothing. Well, almost nothing. Try relaxation.

Get in a comfortable sitting position, maintaining your breathing in a normal way. Close your eyes and repeat a favorite word or phrase, perhaps simply "one" or "relaxing". Repeat this word over and over again pushing all other thoughts and stimuli out of your mind.

Concentrate on this one word and clear your mind of all else for five minutes, saying your key word over and over again in your mind. Try hard not to go to sleep during this exercise.

Dr. Herb Benson of Boston calls this procedure "the relaxation response."

This technique is similar to many of the world's religious prayer rituals, and is almost identical to the transcendental meditation with the exception that the one key word replaces the mantra or the prayer.

> **TAME THE PAIN TIP**
>
> *Try placing a pillow under your knees when you lie down. This may help relieve the pressure on your sciatic nerve reducing your pain.*

Will it work for you? Nobody claims to know all the benefits of this type of relaxation response, but most experts agree that it can reduce stress and in many cases reduce the severity of pain. Some think that such a regimen helps the brain and the spinal cord to release endorphins that are known to help relax and bring about a state of well-being. Endorphins are natural painkillers and thought to be the body's naturally produced version of morphine.

Biofeedback

This method of pain relief is not as popular as it was only a few years ago however many users still swear by it and it is certainly worth mentioning. The purpose of biofeedback in the case of back pain is to help regulate posture and movement and release muscle tension and pain.

Biofeedback uses a computer linked to sensors on the body that provide video and audio readouts of your muscular reactions. The tension in your muscles, the temperature of your fingers and the amount of sweat you produce can all be used to show areas of muscle tension.

You are taught to relax the muscle as a voluntary and controlled response to the feedback. When this works, the relaxed muscle can result in a reduction of your pain.

Hydrotherapy

Some doctors and homeopaths advise the use of hydrotherapy as a means of reducing the inflammation associated with sciatica and in many cases reducing the pain. Most people think of exercising in a heated pool as hydrotherapy but any therapeutic use of water is actually hydrotherapy.

Hot and Cold Compresses

Take two towels, large enough to be folded to three times and cover the affected area you want to treat, in this case your lower back. Soak one towel in hot tap water and wring it out, fold into three thicknesses and apply to your back or have someone else put on the towel while you're lying on your stomach.

Leave this towel in place for three minutes. During that time take the second towel and soak it in cold tap water or ice water. Wring it out. Replace the hot towel after three minutes with the cold one for a minute. Now soak the hot towel again and repeat the rotation of hot and cold. This procedure can be done for twenty to thirty minutes to help relieve the pain and promote healing.

How does it work? The hot towel heats up and expands all of the capillaries in the affected area, which at once draws more blood than usual into the heated area. The blood helps to repair any damage to the spinal area and fight inflammation. Then the cold towel comes and drives the blood away. A minute later the hot towel comes and fresh blood surges into the area.

This infusion of new blood every minute or so will help your back to heal and to reduce the pain.

Other forms of hydrotherapy include hot/cold showers, and a warm bath. Don't let the bath be too hot or it will reduce the effect. You can also use Epsom salts in a warm bath or various herbs for an herbal bath.

Acupuncture

Acupuncture has been practiced in China for over 5,000 years. It came to the United States in the 1970's with a bang and held a lot of popular appeal, but then it faded and almost died out. Now it has been Westernized and many medical doctors and specialists use it in their regular practice.

Acupuncture is the placement of needles into what are called acupuncture points where the Chinese say the blood and bodily energy converge. Western doctors who studied this new technique quickly discovered that the 800 Chinese points correspond roughly with the western physicians understanding of the neural structures. This meant that Western doctors could use their understanding of the neural points as the basis for acupuncture treatments. They did not have to study the Chinese system and learn a whole new set of 800 points on the human body. Now a Western physician could utilize acupuncture as part of a treatment using Western medical principles and choosing the points for the needles on an anatomical basis.

Needles. The very idea gives some people the impulse to run screaming for the woods. But you should be aware that the needles used in acupuncture are extremely thin, rounded on the end, and unlike needles used to give shots of medication they do not need to be hollow. This makes them, in most cases virtually pain free.

Certain treatments may produce a stinging bug bite type feeling, but usually the doctor or therapist knows this ahead of time and will let you know exactly what to expect. Also remember with a shot, much of the pain comes not from the needle, but from the solution being injected into your body.

The traditional method of using needles, still widely practiced, is to insert them at the proper place and then twirl them. Now some users employ a device that will twirl the needles and at the same time electrically stimulate the area. This is called electroacupuncture and does not hurt, rather it gives the patient a pulsating feeling.

There are two theories about how acupuncture works. The older one is that the needles stimulate the large nerve fibers, which send sensations such as temperature and touch to the brain. The smaller nerve fibers send the pain signals to the brain.

The theory is that the large fibers are over-stimulated until they overload. Somehow this overload acts as a valve that also shuts down the small nerve fibers in the area. If the nerve can't send the pain signal to the brain, the patient doesn't feel the pain.

The other theory is that the human brain can produce powerful painkillers called endorphins and enkephalins. Some experts say that the use of acupuncture will stimulate the brain to produce these two natural opiate painkillers.

The idea is that the acupuncture stimulates one specific area and the brain gets the message and quickly sends endorphins by way of the nervous system back to the spot where the acupuncture was given. This then turns off the pain and the patient feels better.

Does it work? That you'll have to figure out for yourself through trial and error. If nothing else seems to satisfy your pain reduction needs, give acupuncture a try. It can't hurt anything.

Will it work on sciatica? One patient had serious sciatica pain and could find no relief. She

GOOD TO KNOW

One study, published in the CLINICAL JOURNAL OF PAIN, gave further evidence of the successful use of acupuncture for the relief of back pain.

Fifty participants who had been suffering with lower back pain for at least six months and had tried a variety of other treatments before were divided into three groups, a traditional acupuncture group, an electroacupuncture group and a placebo group. Patients were treated once per week for eight weeks with 20-minute sessions with the placebo group receiving mock stimulations. A follow-up treatment was given 2 months later, and a final treatment was given after two more months.

Throughout the study patients kept a pain journal in which they recorded pain intensity, use of pain medications, sleep quality, and activity levels. In addition an independent observer who was not aware of what types of acupuncture the different groups were receiving made regular assessments of the patients based on clinical interviews and physical examinations.

Analysis of the pain diaries and independent assessments revealed what researchers deemed "significant" difference in the pain relief recorded by the acupuncture recipients and the placebo group. Those that received acupuncture showed lower than baseline morning and evening pain scores as well as an overall decrease of reported pain throughout the duration of the study. The placebo group by contrast had higher than baseline pain scores that remained elevated over baseline for the duration of the study. Activity levels were also increased in the acupuncture group and sleep disturbances were much lower than the placebo group as well.

went to an acupuncturist who was also a medical doctor. He used ten different sized needles from one to three inches long. Two were inserted on each side of the spine near the point where the L5 vertebra nerve roots come out of the spinal canal. Two more went in at the S2 area with one on each side of the spine.

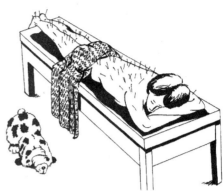

The other six needles were positioned down the left leg of the woman where she felt the intense sciatica pain. The needles were stimulated with electrical current. After the first thirty-minute treatment she felt better. After four treatments a week apart, the sciatica pain was almost gone.

Acupuncture is not a mysterious end-all for pain. It may not completely stop a pain, but many medicines don't completely stop pain either.

Some states have strict laws regarding acupuncture while other states are more lenient. You may wish to check the legal ramifications in your area before contacting an acupuncturist. One rule of thumb: if there are ads for acupuncturists in your local telephone yellow pages, they are probably legal and licensed in your area. See Appendix II at the end of this book for some reliable acupuncture information and referral resources.

Acupressure

Acupressure is the fraternal twin to acupuncture. Basically the only difference is that acupressure uses finger and hand pressure on the pressure points of the body instead of the needles of acupuncture.

Thumb pressure is done with the ball of the thumb. The thrust is perpendicular to the pressure point. It can be a back and forth method or a circular motion with the side of the thumb and nail.

Other techniques include the use of finger pressure, grasping skin between finger and thumb, tapping a pressure point with fist, knuckle, palm or finger, rubbing, clenched fist rocking and the pinching of flesh.

Acupressure is thought to work by breaking the reflex arc between the pressure points just beneath the skin and those various organs to which it communicates. It rearranges the forces of the body that channel pain and hurt in a part of the body. This tends to sedate the automatic nervous system that was complaining, and a more normal state is achieved.

- Acupressure increases the flow of arterial blood.

- Acupressure stimulates the endocrine gland.

- Acupressure stimulates lymph gland and venous drainage.

- Acupressure releases waste products from musculature.

- Acupressure helps to produce physiological peace and mental relaxation.

- Acupressure lowers the pain and the hurting.

This isn't intended to be a course in acupressure. Whole books are written on it. For example there are over 200 pressure points on the body you'll need to know about (or your therapist will), eight on the face alone.

How does acupressure apply to sciatica and other back pain? For sciatica, acupressure regimens call for searching for hypersensitive points in these locations:

- middle of the thigh

- in the sciatic notch of the pelvic bones

- at the fifth lumbar vertebra

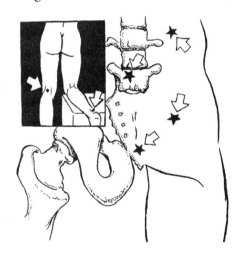

Figure 6:
Acupressure for pain relief in the lower back tends to concentrate on several specific pressure points.

- the crest of the ileum in back

- at the outside of the ankle bones

- in the popliteal space behind the knee

Now, to treat for sciatica pain in the lower back, the buttocks and the legs and ankles, apply finger or thumb pressure at these points:

- At the crest of the ileum on your back.

- In the sciatic notch in the pelvic bones.

- In the middle of the thigh.

- In the popliteal space behind the knee.

- At the outside anklebones.

Now, for the second sequence of treatment for your sciatica pain use acupressure on this trigger point:

- At the fifth lumbar vertebra.

The important element in this treatment is to find relief from the pain. The second action should be to find the source of the problem. Otherwise no matter how good your treatment the pain will come back.

Acupressure can't be detailed properly in a short description such as this. For further information about it consult one of various books on the subject at your library or a holistic store. You may also find books on acupressure at a large bookstore or find an acupressure specialist in your area.

Reflexology

Reflexology is a technique for reducing tension and promoting well-being. It is entirely non-invasive and works on many of the same principles as acupuncture and acupressure. Reflexology deals with the use of hand pressure on specific parts of the hands and feet only. A reflexology chart of the reflex points in the foot is similar in many ways to a chart in an acupuncture manual showing the foot's pressure points.

Reflexology is said to be a completely safe form of therapy besides being a relaxing and pleasant experience. The purpose of reflexology is to normalize the body's functioning, to help break down tension and stress. It also can improve nerve functioning and increase the blood supply all through the body.

Reflexology strives to correct three factors in the body: congestion, inflammation and tension. The reflexology experts say that congestion can lead to growths in the body. Inflammation can show up in conditions such as colitis and sinusitis. Tension can lead to an overall lowering of the efficiency of the immune system.

To create these benefits, reflexology is intended to improve the body's circulation and to help it by speeding up the elimination of waste products and toxins. Reflexology is also said to stimulate the release of endorphins to help control the perception of pain.

Proponents say that reflexology works the best when it is used for the whole body, not for a specific pain or problem. That way it improves the entire body's function, which helps with the natural healing processes where they are needed.

Reflexology for Sciatica

Begin by supporting the right foot with the right hand and use the index and third fingers of your left hand to work up the area just behind the ankle for about three inches. Repeat this pressure treatment three times. Then change feet and do the same thing on the left foot supporting it with the left hand and using the right hand for the application of pressure.

The procedure should continue with treatments for the hips and pelvis. Do this by holding the right foot in an outward direction with your left hand. Use four fingers of your right hand to massage around the edge of the heel forward and then down. Repeat this pressure three times, then move to the other foot and repeat the process.

For hand reflexology for the spine do this: For the reflex points for your spine on your right hand, work along the line from the base of your thumb, straight across the bottom of your hand, then up the length of your thumb. Do this three times for no more than seven seconds each. Repeat the pressure on your left hand.

For treatment for the spinal area on the foot: Hold the top of the right foot with your left hand. Then use your right thumb to work up the reflex points along the right side of the bottom of the foot all the way to the big toe. Repeat three times, then do the other foot the same way.

Reflexology is not an exact science. What might help one person may not affect another at all. Again whole books are written on this subject. For further reading in the field, contact your local library or a bookstore. Also see Appendix II at the back of this book.

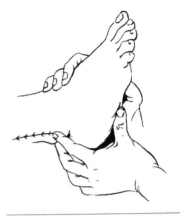

Figure 7:
To treat the spine area spots on the right foot are often stimulated.

Chiropractic

Millions of people worldwide utilize the services of chiropractors to help them with physical problems. Chiropractic uses the knowledge of the nerve functions of the body in conjunction with the laws of anatomy and physiology to help produce normal nerve functions through the spinal column.

> **TAME THE PAIN TIP**
>
> When you have to stand for long periods of time be sure to shift your weight from foot to foot. If possible rest one leg on a step or stool alternating legs periodically.

Many of the chiropractors of today are well-educated persons with six years of study behind them including a year of internship in a chiropractic facility. Their specialty is the spine. Their basic tool of operation is the manipulation of the spine.

A chiropractor is not permitted to prescribe drugs or any prescription medications. He can't draw blood or do any invasive procedures. Chiropractors can order X-rays taken and evaluate them. They can also utilize ultrasound treatments.

For years there has been a conflict between the chiropractors and the medical doctors. The chiropractors say the doctors are drug pushers and slicers and cutters. The medical doctors say the chiropractors try to make differential diagnoses of the back and back pain without adequate training, examination skills, knowledge or experience.

Manipulation

The therapeutic mainstay of those who call themselves chiropractors is manipulation. This has been described as "an assisted passive motion applied to the spinal facet joints and sacroiliac joints."

An expert put it his way. "There's a stiff joint and you manipulate it and that makes it move. This increases the range of motion. A mobile joint is less likely to be painful than a stiff joint."

The key here is "Range Of Motion", or ROM. Near the end of a joint's normal physiological range of motion is a buffer zone. Next to that is an elastic shield. This fiber shield has a spring like feel which a negative pressure inside the joint's capsule creates. This pressure helps stabilize a joint.

When the parts of a joint are pressured beyond this elastic shield by manipulation, they come apart with a cracking sound. This is manipulation. The cracking is caused by the sudden escape of gases inside the synovial fluid of the joint's capsule. Another word for it is cavitation. Such bubbles of gas can be seen on an X-ray right after manipulation. They are usually absorbed within 30 minutes.

For that time, the elastic shield between the buffer zone and the paraphysiological ROM is not there. This leaves more room in the joint space and that makes the joint unstable. No more manipulation of this joint is safe. After the gases are absorbed back into the joint, it becomes normal again.

As in any profession, there are all shades and types of chiropractors. Some guarantee you the moon making great claims of success. Others are more conservative. One chiropractor says he'd rather treat people with sudden back pain than those with chronic pain. He says he can adjust a patient's back that has chronic back pain and he'll feel great for twenty minutes, but then the patient is right back where he was.

On the other hand, with a person who has made a sudden wrong move and has a fixated or frozen joint, a chiropractor can really help. After the inflammation has gone down, such a joint many times remains frozen. This chiropractor says his treatments help unfreeze the joint and the patient is back to normal.

Some chiropractors imply that their manipulation may also affect diseases of internal organs. Is this justified? Most experts agree that manipulation can accelerate the body's blood flow and heart rate. However beyond that there is no evidence that supports the idea that manipulation can have any affect whatsoever on general health or any visceral pathology, diseases or conditions.

SOME WARNING SIGNS OF A POOR TO BAD CHIROPRACTOR

- If he insists on taking X-rays of your full spine.

- If he fails to take a complete medical history and do a clinical examination before beginning treatment.

- If he claims the treatment will improve your immune function or cure a disease.

- If he tries to get other family members to begin treatments with him.

- If he insists that you sign a contract for long-term care.

- If he promises to prevent disease through regular checkups or manipulation.

- If he promises to prevent back pain through regular treatments.

- If he suggests that chiropractic can be viewed as a primary health care function.

Another problem many people find with chiropractors is their programs that call for preventive manipulation of patients when they are pain free. The extended plans of patient care that include twelve and up to twenty-four visits for treatment of an out of alignment spine are also looked upon by many in the medical community as a money wasting over-treatment by fast talking chiropractors.

The Role of the Medical Doctor

One major concern of medical doctors is that when a patient is treated by a chiropractor the patient is getting only a partial diagnosis of any potential problems. Most chiropractors are not trained to make a diagnosis of all of the factors that might be producing a symptom.

Most doctors suggest that after you see your chiropractor, you also see your family doctor to check further for other complications from your back pain or other causes. There are several serious medical problems that can radiate pain into the back or down the arm that have nothing to do with either the back or the arm.

This is what worries medical doctors. They say such diseases that can be missed by chiropractors looking at back pain include an expanding aortic aneurysm, angina, paget's disease, goiter or a thyroid problem.

Many of today's better-trained chiropractors agree with the idea that they should work in conjunction with medical doctors to be sure that all of the potential causes of a problem can be investigated.

So Will Manipulation Help Your Sciatica?

It might and it might not. There are four main ways that many experts say manipulation could affect your back pain:

- Manipulation can improve the mobility between two vertebrae, which will reduce the temporary inflammation that happens as a result of a locked spinal joint.

- Manipulation can help the smaller spinal muscles attaching one vertebra to another to relax which can reduce spasming and the pain that accompanies it.

- Manipulation can reduce the nerve irritation as a result of the improved mobility of the vertebra.

- Manipulation can cause the body to increase the release of endorphins, the body's natural painkiller, which can help relieve the pain of sciatica.

Chiropractors typically do not do any manipulations if their examination or X-rays show that there is any evidence of bone fractures, infection, cancer, severe arthritis or other possible conditions that would be aggravated by manipulation.

To manipulate or not to manipulate. It's up to you. The controversy continues. A middle of the road approach might be to try chiropractic if nothing else is working after you've seen your medical doctor.

On the other side if you see a chiropractor first and get treatments, follow up with a visit to your GP or specialist medical doctor to be sure you have all of the medical bases covered including those that the chiropractor can't evaluate.

There is lots of anecdotal evidence for the use of chiropractic to reduce back pain. Thousands of people will swear to its successful use in their case. However unlike some other alternative treatments this one, according to some doctors, could cause damage if done incorrectly. So if you are interested in chiropractic just be sure to choose your chiropractor carefully. See Appendix II at the back of the book for some organizations that may be of some help in this area.

Yoga

Many people have heard of Yoga but have no real idea what it is all about. Some think of it as a mystical excursion into an incense-laden room with a long bearded guru smiling and meditating with them.

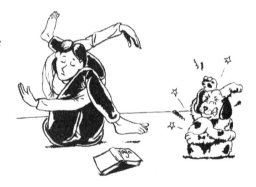

Well folks, yoga has totally gone mainstream and while you certainly can still find some incense-laden yoga sessions these days you can also practice yoga in a brightly lit gymnasium at the local YMCA. One of the most popular forms of yoga today is hatha yoga. This is simply a regimen of assuming specific postures and at the same time using proper breathing techniques. With this type of yoga there is no meditation, mental detachment or a search for spiritual growth.

Yoga exercises and breathing techniques have been used for hundreds of years to treat back pain. Yoga began over 4000 years ago in India and has taken a number of different paths and developments to those types of yoga found today. Other types include raja, tantra and jana yoga that do work with meditation and spiritual growth.

The yoga teacher usually works closely with each student on an individual basis to help correct any posture problems. Yoga has a system of postures called asanas. Along with these postures the teacher will work with the student to develop breath control, which is called pranayama.

Many back problems can result from poor posture, stress and structural imbalances. Yoga enthusiasts say that learning even the simplest postures can teach people to see how they distribute their weight, how they use or abuse their spines, and show up any weak points they have in general posture.

TAME THE PAIN TIP

Yoga can help you build your core muscles, those muscles that surround your middle front and back. By strengthening your back and abdominal muscles you help your body to maintain a proper upright posture placing less stress on your spine and possibly reducing or eliminating future back pain.

The breathing aspect is a little more difficult for people to understand. Yoga teaches that there is a direct connection between people's emotions and how they breathe. Feelings such as hatred, fear, grief even anger can cause physical tension as well as emotional upsets.

By practicing proper breathing techniques while doing the proper posture exercises, a yoga student can learn to have some control over how his or her emotions affect the physical side.

Now, what about that back pain? In yoga the spine is the center of the body, and all postural exercises focus on the spine. The biggest emphasis is lengthening the spine and realigning it. After this has been accomplished through the postures and correct breathing, a lot of a person's back pains will simply go away.

By aligning, the yoga people mean that the human body is in a straight line as if a plumb line were placed on the shoulder and the line would go through the hips and into the ankles in a straight line.

So far we haven't said anything that yoga can do to help out your sciatica. True. Part of the reason you have that herniated or pushed out disc could be your poor posture over the years. The benefit here is that after the disc is healed and the pain gone, you can take up yoga to help keep your back from causing you any more trouble.

In many regimens today, flexibility is considered equally important for the back as exercises that promote strength. With increased flexibility and range of movements, a person can maintain better posture and help avoid all kinds of back problems.

Hypnosis

Can hypnosis help you with your sciatica pain? The answer is a cautious "it can" but it all depends on you—the one hurting.

Hypnosis comes from the Greek word hypnos, meaning to sleep. Most hypnotists these days say that hypnotism is a sleeplike condition physically induced in which the subject loses consciousness but responds with certain limitations to the suggestions of the hypnotist.

You've heard about the nightclub hypnotist who puts unsuspecting guests under hypnosis and then suggests that they do outrageous and embarrassing things on signal after they come out of their trance. This is not the kind of hypnosis we're talking about. Experts say people will not do anything under hypnosis that they wouldn't want to do without the hypnosis and will do nothing against their personal code of ethics.

Some experts say that hypnosis is when a person is in an altered state of awareness when the subject focuses on one subject and screens out all the rest. This lets the one hypnotized to get in touch with his or her subconscious and utilize it to help work out problems or control conditions.

One professional in the field says that hypnotism is only an acceleration of a natural tendency that we all have: the ability to screen out background noises and situations when we are totally concentrating on one idea, or project. For example a student cramming for a test might not hear the telephone ringing right beside her on the desk.

One of the goals of hypnotism for a sciatica pain patient is to help the patient to change the way the pain is perceived and how it is responded to. If the pain can be labeled as "background" to the patient, it will help him or her to downgrade it and screen it out. Then they can go about other activities without the hurt of the background sciatica.

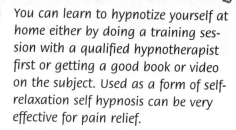

TAME THE PAIN TIP

You can learn to hypnotize yourself at home either by doing a training session with a qualified hypnotherapist first or getting a good book or video on the subject. Used as a form of self-relaxation self hypnosis can be very effective for pain relief.

Hypnotism does not cure sciatica. It can't repair or heal a damaged disc. It can't make your back pain go away. However, hypnotism for many people can do more to relieve sciatic pain and other back pains than a bottle full of pain pills.

So, every time your sciatica kicks up with a thunderbolt of pain do you tear down to your hypnotist for a session? You could, but that would soon make you dependent on your hypnotist and run up your bills. Most hypnotists say it's a simple process for a person to learn how to hypnotize himself.

Hypnosis is good way to help control pain and stress and is recommended by the American Psychiatric Association. It has been used to treat everything from back pain to labor pain.

In some cases, those who use hypnotherapy report that they have better results in controlling pain, fatigue and poor sleep patterns than they have had with physical therapy.

There are three main stages of hypnosis:

Stage one: The first stage of hypnosis is the lightest, sometimes called a superficial trance, in this stage you remain totally aware of your surroundings.

Stage two: The second stage of hypnosis is often called an alpha state. At this stage your breathing becomes more relaxed and slowed and your blood pressure and heart rate drop down. This is the stage that most hypnotherapists will use to work on your pain.

Stage three: This is the deepest level of hypnosis sometimes used by psychiatrist to sharpen faded memories or deal with severe traumas.

One of the best times to try hypnotherapy is when nothing else is working, or high doses of drugs are needed to get the desired pain relief. But be aware that up to 10% of the population cannot apparently be hypnotized.

If the idea of hypnotism appeals to you, you can get more information on hypnosis, or find a qualified licensed hypnotist by visiting the website of the National Guild of Hypnotists at www.ngh.net. You can also learn to hypnotize yourself either by doing a training session with a qualified hypnotherapist first or getting a good book or video on the subject. Used as a form of self-relaxation self hypnosis can be very effective for pain relief.

Don't worry about getting "stuck" in a hypnotic trance. You've seen hypnotists bring subjects out of a trance in movies or on the stage. A person can come out of a trance by himself quickly and easily just by wanting to, or giving a self time limit of three or four minutes.

Homeopathy

This form of homeopathic medicine is not as popular as it once was in the United States, but proponents say it is growing rapidly worldwide. The basic thrust here is that the patient is treated and not the disease. The homeopathic philosophy is that very small qualities of age-old healing substances are used as medicine.

Natural remedies made from animal, vegetable and mineral substances are used and the entire group consists of about 600 medications. The average medical doctor has over 10,000 drugs to choose from.

Homeopathic medications have such small amounts of drugs in them such as belladonna made from the deadly nightshade plant, that they are non-toxic. Homeopathic medications are exempt from most of the Federal Drug Administration control since they contain such small amounts of drugs and medications. However if some homeopathic medication claims it can "cure cancer or AIDS" the FDA will pounce on them and make them prove it. Also, vague claims like, "for immune deficiency problems", will bring action by the FDA. For the most part the FDA has a hands-off policy on homeopathic medications.

In the past, the homeopathic physician almost always prescribed one medicine at a time. This was because the remedy had been tested one at a time on humans, and there was no way to know how a combination of remedies would affect the patient. Now, however, many medicines for sale over the counter in health food stores and those that specialize in homeopathic medications, offer those with several ingredients.

Homeopathy goes by three principles:

1. The law of similarities. The idea here is that the patient's symptoms are studied carefully, and a medication is prescribed that exactly fits these symptoms. The idea is that the same substance that causes the symptoms cures a disease. Hippocrates wrote in 400 B.C. "Through the like, disease is produced and through the application of the like, it is cured." This is called the law of similarities.

2. The law of proving. This deals with the method of testing the remedies. A group of healthy persons is given a remedy. Some get placebo pills in a double blind test. The symptoms of each are carefully recorded. Those who got the remedy and have similar symptoms are written up in the Materia Medica book. This is the physician's reference book. If the symptoms are all the same, the remedy is then used to cure any sick person with the same symptoms.

3. The law of potentization. This refers to the way the remedies are prepared. They are made by a succession of dilutions and shakings and in some cases grinding, until the original sub-

stance has been diluted six times. The higher the dilution, the greater the potency.

Homeopathic medicines are extremely low priced compared to a regular pharmaceutical. A bottle of pills might cost $1.25 instead of $40 to $50 at your local drug store. Why? The five hundred to six hundred most used medications in the homeopathic medicine shelf have been there for the last one hundred and fifty years. Most are inexpensive to produce, none of them is patented, none is the result of a hundred million dollar research and development program at some monolithic pharmaceutical company. All are in the public domain. Neither is there a huge advertising budget to sell the drugs to the public or to the homeopathic practitioners, the cost of which would be passed on to the consumer.

Homeopathic physicians say there is another difference between them and the allopath doctors. The homeopath spends much more time with their patients, getting to know them as individuals, sensing their moods and personalities as well as the problem they are having. They need to know this because often the mood of the patient is one of the symptoms of the ailment. Kind of reminds you of the good old-fashioned common sense country doctor of yesteryear doesn't it?

Will homeopathy help you get rid of your sciatica pain? It can't hurt. None of the homeopathic medications is toxic in any way. A child could gobble up a whole bottle of pills and suffer almost no bad effects. So, if it can't hurt, and it might help there is no harm in trying.

Osteopathy

Back in the late 1800's osteopathy was developed as basically a system of health care that highlighted the central role of the musculoskeletal system in health and disease and the use of spinal manipulation, the bending, twisting and stretching the spine, as a therapy.

Today the Dr. of Osteopathy, D.O., receives a scientific and medical training similar to M.D.'s, and in some states they function in hospitals and clinics and in private practice side by side with the M.D.'s. They generally take four years of college and four years of medical school and a year of internship at an osteopathic hospital. They may go on to take additional training in fields such as rheumatology and orthopedic surgery, however most don't. About 90 percent of D.O.'s are in family practice.

Doctors of Osteopathy generally tend to use fewer drugs and less surgery and opt instead for non-invasive methods as well as manipulation to help patients regain or maintain their health.

> **TAME THE PAIN TIP**
>
> *Light back exercises and walking briskly on grassy ground or on a sandy beach is kinder to your back than running or jogging on concrete or asphalt roads or footpaths.*

Osteopathy and Sciatica

The D.O. will usually take a detailed history about your pain and your past medical history. Then a palpatory examination is made. This is a gentle tactile use of his fingers to test the tissue tone and mobility around the pain area. A physical examination will be done and X-rays taken when necessary. The osteopath physician says this will enable him or her to either confirm or rule out the protruding or ruptured disc as the cause of the pain.

If it is a disc at fault, the D.O. will then use manipulative therapy to ease the pressure on the disc, and then with gentle exercise and care, the slow repair can take place. In extreme cases surgery may be needed to remove any extruded pulp from the disc.

For help defining sciatica trouble, there are some reflex centers that osteopaths, as well as other doctors, check for considerable soreness. If they find it, this usually indicates a sciatica condition. These are at the front of the body and called ropy contractions, which indicate lymphatic congestion associated with sciatic pain down one or both legs. These three points are:

- A ropy point that starts one-fifth the distance below the large bony protuberance of the upper leg bone and on for a distance of 50 to 90 millimeters downwards on the back outer part of the upper leg bone.

- A ropy point starting one fifth the distance above the knee and continuing upward for a matter of 50 millimeters on the back outer part of the upper leg bone.

- A ropy point in the mid-back area of the upper leg bone and one-third of the distance upward from the knee joint.

Osteopaths would rather have you prevent back trouble and sciatica than have to cure it. They have developed a given set of exercises for you to do to help insure good back health. These will be covered in Chapter 7 of the book.

State licenses and regulations vary from state to state concerning the practices of doctors of osteopathy. In some states they are on par with M.D.'s and work in and through hospitals and with insurance companies. In other states they are more restricted. Check for the availability and areas of operation in your state.

Orthopaedic Physicians

Don't confuse this group of M.D.'s with orthopedic surgeons. The orthopaedic physician is a specialist in soft tissue especially of the back. He works with injuries to the discs, muscles, ligaments, tendons, joint capsules and other soft tissue of the back that can't be evaluated by X-rays or myelograms.

Orthopaedic medicine is the "nonsurgical management of soft tissue disorders of the musculoskeletal system. Surgery for ailments of the musculoskeletal system should remain within the domain of the orthopaedic surgeon."

The orthopaedic physician locates non-bone problems, such as the cause of sciatic pain, by using a six major movements test: flexion, extension, right rotation, left rotation, right side flexion and left side flexion. First the patient does each one by himself. Then the same motions are repeated but the patient remains passive, the muscles don't contract and the doctor can tell where the pain is coming from.

The last test is when the patient does the same motions against resistance, which means the doctor can tell if there is pain, and whether it's coming from a muscle or a tendon.

Usually if five or fewer of the motions result in pain, the doctors check for a protruding disc. This is not the extreme disc problem that orthopaedic surgeons can find with a myelogram. These will be the smaller problems called a soft disc problem or a hard disc problem.

Many times the soft disc problem can be treated with traction. The hard disc type can often be cured with manipulation. If these don't work and there is still pain, these orthopaedic physicians sometimes use a caudal epidural block. This is an injection of the anesthetic procaine into a specific spot in the back. It goes into the caudal aperture, a small opening in the tailbone. The procaine rises up the spinal canal to the lumbar disc level.

It works, but doctors aren't sure why. Some think that it desensitizes the nerve root and can also hydraulically separate a protruding disc from the nerve root or the dura mater that had caused the pain.

Sometimes one such treatment solves the sciatica or other back pain. Sometimes it might need to be redone every six months to a year.

Orthopaedic physicians are not in competition with orthopaedic surgeons. Actually they complement each other. If you're looking for an orthopaedic physician check with your local medical association.

Supplements and Sciatica

People prone to back problems should consider a supplement program that consists of bone and muscle building supplements as well as inflammation and pain treating supplements.

Vitamins and Minerals

Your body needs vitamins and minerals to function properly. Many of us do not get what we need from our diet. In the case of those of use with back pain there are certain vitamins and minerals we should concentrate on that may be effective in promoting healing and alleviating pain.

Below is a short list of some of the vitamins and minerals you should be sure to include in your diet.

- **Vitamin B complex** helps your body build strong and healthy bones

- **Vitamin C** aids helps repair damaged tissues including those in your muscles, tendons, and bones

- **Vitamin E** is an antioxidant that can help repair tissues including those in your injured back

- **Boron** is important for building strong bones

- **Selenium** aids in building strong bones and muscles including those in the back

- **Magnesium** both helps build muscles and aids in proper muscle functioning

Another combination supplement that some experts recommend is Calcium-Zinc-Magnesium tablets, four daily with vitamin D of 400 IU. Also B complex of 100 mg with extra B-1 of 100 mg, B-6 of 250 mg and niacin of 250 mg.

Valerian Root

Valerian root can be taken as a tea or in tablet or capsule forms. It acts as a mild muscle relaxant and tranquilizer. Some people with back pain find it a very effective sleep-aid helping to relax the back and allow for a restful night's sleep.

Devil's Claw

Devil's Claw can be an effective pain reliever. One German study, consisting of 109 people suffering with low back pain, suggests that in some cases the herb Devil's Claw can relieve back pain. Half of the study participants received a placebo and the other half of the group was given Devil's Claw. All participants were also allowed to take any prescription pain relievers they were on as needed during the course of the study. After one month nine in the Devil's Claw group were reportedly pain free while only one in the placebo group was pain free.

Chamomile

You may already be familiar with the relaxing effect of chamomile tea. Chamomile acts as a mild muscle relaxant and tranquilizer. It can be taken before bed to help relieve muscle tension and stress that can keep you from getting a good night's sleep.

Bromelain

Bromelain is a natural enzyme found in pineapples. Some people find that this enzyme is effective at reducing swelling and inflammation. It may help reduce your back pain.

TAME THE PAIN TIP

Black cohosh, a member of the buttercup family, is an herbal used to treat a variety of troubling pain related symptoms. The root of this plant has shown some promise as a mild sedative and anti-inflammatory and so may be useful in addressing sciatica pain. Other herbals that have shown some pain reliving characteristics are white willow bark, devil's claw, and flaxseed oil. If you choose to try white willow bark be sure to check with your doctor first to make sure it will not interact with any other pain relievers you may be taking.

Diet and Sciatica

Some dietary experts say that diet can have an influence on sciatica and that if sciatica sufferers pay more attention to what they eat it can make a difference in their pain. A healthy eating plan can help ward off gas and digestion problems which can contribute to back troubles as well as give your body the nutrients it needs to build healthy strong muscles and bones.

Intestinal Gas and Digestive Problems

Having excess intestinal gas or other digestive problems can affect your back. Since the intestines are close to the back a build up of gas and toxins can affect your back and even lead to pain in the back.

Following are some tips for avoiding digestive woes:

■ be sure to chew up your food thoroughly

- eat slowly

- sit down to eat

- avoid drinking to many carbonated drinks

- avoid drinking to much coffee

- limit animal protein, the hardest to digest

- eat a fiber rich diet to avoid constipation and the build up of gas

- drink plenty of water to avoid constipation

Eat Your Fruits and Vegetables

Your body uses the simple sugars found in fruit as fuel to run including keeping your muscles, nerves, and bones in tip-top shape. The vitamins, minerals, water and fiber in fruits and vegetables all contribute to a healthy body and a healthy back. Make sure you get plenty of them in your diet. You should be eating at least two servings of each a day.

TAME THE PAIN TIP

A surprising way to help avoid sciatic pain is to make sure you are eating a well balanced diet including lots of high fiber foods, fruits, and vegetables. Turns out that straining to have a bowel movement when you are constipated might lead to a flare up of sciatic pain.

Bad-Back Juice Fast

Following is a specific week long sciatica diet that begins with a juice fast. The diet is to be used when you have a bad flare up. It emphasizes alkaline foods that should counteract the tissue acidity in your inflamed sciatica.

Day One:

- Start with a glass of hot water mixed with the juice of half a lemon.

- For breakfast a glass of freshly made juice from apple, grape, carrot, orange or pineapple.

- Half way through the morning, take a glass of mineral water with a slice of lemon in it.

- Your lunch consists of only a glass of juice similar to what you had for breakfast. Make sure it's fresh squeezed or blended.

- Break up your afternoon with another glass of water and that lemon slice.

- For dinner you get another glass of pure juice with a teaspoon of vegetable concentrate, yeast extract or concentrated apple juice.

Day Two:

- Repeat the menu for day one being careful to use only fresh juices sticking to the citrus. No bananas.

Day Three:

- As soon as you get up have a glass of fruit juice or hot cider vinegar and honey drink.

- Breakfast this day is fresh fruit salad with a quarter cup of sunflower seeds.

- For your midmorning pickup, try herbal tea, or a favorite juice.

- For lunch fix a raw salad from vegetables, and add a baked potato and baked onion. Add cheese or milled nuts.

- Afternoon break have a cup of herbal tea.

- Dinner is a mixed raw salad or a mixed vegetable stew or broth.

- Before bedtime take another juice drink.

Days Four to Seven:

- Breakfast is a baked apple with raisins or fresh fruit.

- Break: herbal tea or fruit juice.

- Lunch: Raw salad with dressing, fresh fruit cup sprinkled with wheat germ.

■ Dinner: Raw salad and dressing, vegetable broth, fresh fruit or baked apple or dried prunes.

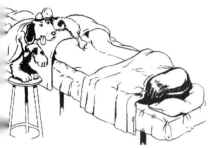

Chapter Five:

Treating Sciatica with Surgery

While there are many causes for back pain there are really only two that can be treated successfully with surgery.

If an MRI or a CAT scan shows clearly that you have a herniated disc or one bulging out so much that it is giving you constant sciatica pain, that is one of the types of back conditions that can be operated on. The procedure is called a discotomy, and means that the injured disc that is pressing a nerve is partially removed.

The other type of surgery for back pain is called stabilization and involves fusing two or more vertebrae together. This might be needed for a variety of reasons but one would be where a vertebra is cracked and this allows the vertebra to actually slip forward in relation to the vertebra below. This can cause terrible pain from pressure on the nerve roots. The problem is called spondylolisthesis.

These are the two major types of operations surgeons perform to help relieve back pain. There are a few other operations done for spine trauma, infection or a tumor, but an estimated ninety-five percent of all back operations are of these two types.

Today slightly more than ninety percent of all of you with back pain will never have surgery for it. You simply could not possibly be helped by such back surgery.

To be a good candidate for surgery your back pain must not respond to any other kind of treatment. Then it must be specific and the surgeon must be able to pinpoint the problem.

There is no way that even the best surgeon can help you if your back problems are caused by serious wear and tear of the spine and the discs over a long period of time.

Decompression Surgery

The most common type of decompression surgery is a discotomy in which part of the offending disc is simply removed. Usually the doctor has to cut away a small portion of bone on the vertebra to be able to get to the herniated or bulging disc.

The surgery takes about an hour and starts with a two-inch incision in the lower back. The surgeon pushes in and around the various muscles and ligaments. Usually there must be a piece of bone cut away to gain access to the problem disc. Doctors call this procedure a laminectomy.

In a discotomy the whole disc is not removed. Once in the right place, the surgeon enlarges the existing hole in the disc's outer wall and scoops out most of the soft nucleus. This eliminates the pressure on the nerve and stops the pain. Then the surgeon moves the nerve root, ligaments and muscles back in place and stitches up the incision.

If a piece of bone is irritating a root nerve, it is located by X-ray and then removed much the same way that an offending disc is. The problem bone spur or growth is cut away relieving the pressure on the sciatic nerve root and the pain is eliminated.

The Microdiscotomy

Gaining more favor these days is the microdiscotomy, which is simply the same discotomy but performed with a smaller incision and through a smaller area of the back with the aid of lights and a special operating microscope. The benefits here are that the surgery takes less time, the incision is half the size as usual, there is less loss of blood, less post-operation pain, shorter hospitalization times, quicker return to normal activities and less scar tissue.

While some orthopaedists frown on the smaller operating window and the procedure in general, many think that the micro type operation will be the accepted method in the future.

Spinal Fusion

The other type of surgery performed for sciatica or other back pain is called spinal fusion. This is when two or three vertebrae are fused together so they are motionless to give the back greater stability.

In about a quarter of the cases of decompression surgery, it is necessary to stabilize the affected area because the space between the vertebrae has worn down and is too narrow. This often means there has been too much wear and tear on the resident facet joints. To return the back to a more stable function, the surgeon decides that the fusion needs to take place.

Another time fusion is needed is when spondylolisthesis, the cracking and movement of a vertebra, does not get better with regular and conservative treatments. The cause of this problem is easy to see on an X-ray. Then fusing is needed.

GOOD TO KNOW

A study published in the December 2001 issue of the journal SPINE cast doubts on the success rate if fusion surgery for chronic lower back pain sufferers. Turns out only 1 in 6 of those who had surgery were rated as having an "excellent" result two years after their surgery.

Fusion Surgery

The surgery begins much like that for a discotomy. The incision on the lumbar region is about three inches long because more space inside will be needed. First the surgeon will roughen up the tips of the two facet joints; this will help them to heal better later and to fuse with new bone pieces.

Through another incision, the surgeon takes small strips of bone from the patient's pelvis. These bone strips are an inch long and less than one-sixteenth of an inch thick.

These strips in effect become splints and braces that are packed by the surgeon against the damaged sur-

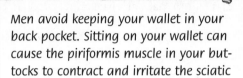

TAME THE PAIN TIP

Men avoid keeping your wallet in your back pocket. Sitting on your wallet can cause the piriformis muscle in your buttocks to contract and irritate the sciatic nerve leading to sciatica flare-ups.

faces of the vertebrae. The body thinks the roughened areas have been broken and it rushes healing material to the site fusing the roughed up vertebrae and the splints into a solid and stable unit, eliminating the pain and giving the spine more strength.

Chymopapain Injections

Chymopapain is an enzyme, derived from the papaya plant, that when injected, in a treatment called Chemonucleolysis, into a herniated disc breaks down the noncollagen components of the nucleus reducing the pressure and pain. Yes, it is invasive, but not nearly so much as even a microdiscotomy.

Chymopapain was approved for use in 1982. More widely used in Europe and Japan the drug was initially viewed with some skepticism by some orthopedic surgeons and neurosurgeons. However three major double-blind studies have shown a success rate with the drug between 71% to 83%.

In spite of its success rate the drug changed hands through five different pharmacuatical companies before in 2002 being discontinued for business reasons. However there is still much interest in the drug and it is likely to make a reappearance on the market in the near future.

Chymopapain and Sciatica

What kind of a patient should be considered for the use of chymopapain? One who has a herniated disc that is compressing a lumbar nerve root. Your typical sciatica sufferer. There should be a CAT scan or a myelogram to pin point a definite disc protrusion. Then the patient should have undergone up to twelve weeks of conservative treatments that have not produced any relief.

Not everyone agrees. Some orthopaedists say that if a patient has had severe sciatic pain for more than two years, a chymopapain injection isn't the best procedure. They say that after two years the spine has made adaptive changes, such as adhesions, that make the problem more complicated than just a herniated disc.

Many doctors report great success with the injections including long-term relief. They point out that since there is no incision, there is no resulting scar tissue, which often leads to problems years later from discotomy patients.

How Chymopapain Works

It is thought that chymopapain acts on the nucleus of a herniated disc in much the same way meat tenderizer does on a tough steak. The injected fluid breaks down the protein material in the nucleus of the disc, but doesn't damage the outer ring, which is made up of cartilage. The nucleus, which has been dissolved into a fluid, is then absorbed by the blood stream and excreted through the urine.

It essentially does the same job as that small scoop the surgeon uses to take out the nucleus in a discotomy. It does it slower but with no cutting of bone or tissue and is a thousand times less invasive.

The Procedure

The procedure is relatively simple. Any orthopaedic surgeon who does diagnostic discogram tests or a radiologist should be able to do chymopapain injections with a little practice. General anesthetic is used and usually the procedure is done in an operating room, although some surgeons prefer to use local anesthesia.

During the procedure X-rays are shown on a fluroscope screen so the six inch long needle can be precisely positioned by the doctor. Then 1.55 cubic centimeters of chymopapain is injected into the herniated disc's nucleus.

That's it. The needle is withdrawn and the patient goes into a recovery room.

Recovery is about the same as for a discotomy. The sciatica pain is usually gone in two to three days.

Side Effects

There have been reported side effects with the drug. Although 87% of the reported side effects occurred in the first two years after the drug was introduced to the market. The most serious side effect is an allergic reaction that can lead to anaphylaxis and even death. Anaphylaxis occurred in only 0.25% of injections. Also, as with any invasive procedure, there are minor risks of hemorrhagic or neurological problems.

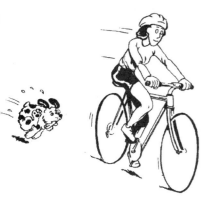

Chapter Six:

Self Help Therapy

Let's get back to basics here. You have back pain. This isn't that ache or mild discomfort you've felt before. Not just a few twinges, but a full blown scream-at-everybody-and-throw-things kind of pain down the back of one or both legs that won't quit when you sit down or lie down or bend over or curl into a ball.

What's first? Most people limp, crawl or slide to a telephone and call the family doctor for a talk and an appointment. If you can get a doctor on the phone these days, most will suggest that you rest and relax for a couple of days and then see how you feel. The M.D. might even suggest some mild pain pills such as Motrin or Advil or Aleve to help you manage the pain.

So, the first step. Many times this two days of lying around and watching old movies and reruns <u>will</u> be enough to make you feel better. A lot of times whatever caused that sharp, burning bright sciatica attack down the backs of your legs will correct itself and the pain will fade, then be gone. Yes, it happens.

All too often though, the pain won't go away and the over the counter pain reliever you are taking isn't doing the job. So you go see your doctor. First he'll ask you a lot of questions, take a history of any back pain and get a physical exam of your back and legs and probably ask you to do some motions with arms and legs. When it's over he'll have a better idea of what's causing your problem.

If he thinks it's sciatica, he may give you some more pain pills and tell you to take it easy for another week, maybe two. Not bed rest but just no heavy lifting or unusual activity. This is the conservative approach to see if the body can heal itself or if there is a problem that needs more medical intervention.

So, we've come to the place where you can do some self help work to see if you can assist in getting your back in shape.

By now you know that if it's a serious herniated disc or a bad protrusion of the disc against a sciatic root nerve, rest and pain pills aren't going to cure you. But you can't be sure that's the diagnosis yet, so it's best to do what you can to help yourself towards recovery.

Pain Pills

These days pain pills come in all sorts of sizes, shapes and potency. Some pills that used to be prescription are now over the counter.

Ibuprofen was a prescription pill for a long time. Now it's available in brand names such as Motrin and Advil and in many plain packaged house brands at major chain drug stores and grocery stores. Buy the house brand. Often they cost half as much as the name brand but they will do exactly what the name brand will do of the same potency. This way you aren't paying for the expensive advertising done by name brands.

Another former prescription pain pill is Aleve, the name brand of naproxen sodium. This is tagged as a pain reliever and fever reducer and comes in at 220 mg for each tablet, but they claim 8 to 12 hours of relief for each two-pill dose. In 2004 Aleve was linked in a NIH study to an increased risk of heart attack and stroke so be sure to discuss its use with your doctor if you are at risk.

Other pills in this pain-relieving category, which are non-prescription and anti-inflammatory, include good old aspirin, like Anacin and Bufferin. You can also get coated varieties of aspirin if it causes stomach upset. These all are non-prescription analgesic and anti-inflammatory.

If you can't take aspirin based pills or ibuprofen, try the acetaminophen non-prescription analgesics like Tylenol. These have no anti-inflammatory properties and can't heal any wounded tissue but they can provide pain relief for some users. Don't use these for more than ten days without consulting your physician.

It might take a little experimenting to find the type of over the counter pain pill that works best for you on your sciatica pain. If you have a favorite for headache or some other pains, the same type of pill will probably work for you on your sciatica, but it might not.

Heat and Cold

If the pain flare-up is a recent occurrence try a cold pack. This might be simply ice cubes in a plastic bag and applying it to your hurting back Be sure to put a cloth or towel between your back and the plastic covered ice cubes. You won't damage your skin that way. Don't keep a cold pack in place for any longer than fifteen-minute intervals.

> ## TAME THE PAIN TIP
>
> To ease sore and tired muscles try this easy at home solution, a microwave heat pack. You will need a tube sock (or a pillowcase or soft cloth), a needle and thread (or sewing machine), and some rice.
>
> - Turn the sock or pillowcase inside out
> - If using cloth sew three side together to form a small bag and turn inside out
> - Fill halfway with rice
> - Sew open end closed
> - Toss in the microwave and turn on high for 2 minutes (test times to find best for you)
> - Wrap your heat pack in a small towel if it's very warm (careful to not make it to hot!)
> - Place on sore spots
> - Reheat as needed
>
> * Note: you should never use heat on a brand new injury

The colder your back gets, the less active the pain nerves will be and you might calm the pain for a time. You aren't curing yourself, just making the pain go away for a while.

A few days after the onset of the pain you should switch to heat. This can be dry heat, such as with a heating pad, or a damp heat with towels soaked in hot water and wrung out. Be sure to protect your skin from the direct heat with a towel. Don't use the hot packs for more than 20 minute at a time intervals. You might also try alternating between cold and hot packs.

The hot packs will bring a flush of new blood into the area. The added blood brings with it white blood cells which can work to help reduce any inflammation and start to repair tissue damage.

Rest Your Back

While rest is recommended for back troubles most doctors these days say that too much bed rest can be bad for your back. The key, as with most things, is moderation. If you took two days of rest after your pain flared up you probably don't need to do it again.

You should however still take things easy until the pain subsides. Finding comfortable restful positions. The important idea here is not to go to work and don't do any lifting or bending to the side. Avoid any activities that might further strain your already hurting back.

Alternative Approaches

Now is the time to take a shot at some of the non-traditional approaches that some people have had sciatica pain relief with. We talked about these in more detail in Chapter Four already, but they are worth repeating. Since at this point you have already been to see your doctor and ruled out any serious issues it is worth giving some of the non-mainstream approaches a try.

You might consider seeing a **chiropractor**. A lot of folks swear by their chiropractors. You've read about them in Chapter Four. Hey, if a chiropractic treatment is going to help your back, the fee for the visit will be worth it. Even if the pain is gone for only a day, it might be worth it for that small island of peace.

Try an **Acupuncturist**. Why not? Those tiny little needles just might overload the major nerves and short stop the small nerves in your sciatica pain area from transmitting any pain. There is enough physical evidence that this works to give acupuncture some credibility. Remember, you have nothing to lose except your pain. Besides, those ultra thin needles don't really hurt.

TAME THE PAIN TIP

When you are in the middle of a sciatica flare-up getting out of bed can be a painful challenge. Done carefully you can avoid further pain. First roll to the side, pull your knees up towards your chest, swing your legs over the side of the bed and push up gently with both arms.

Why not give **hypnosis** a go. Read the section on hypnosis again. It just might work for you. There are a lot of people out there who swear by self-hypnosis for pain relief. There are even clinical studies backing up its use in painful situations like childbirth. So it might be just the ticket for your sciatica pain.

If your pain is not to intense, or perhaps between severe episodes, consider trying **yoga**. While yoga comes in all forms and shapes the kind detailed in the Chapter Four, hatha yoga, might be something that you could do yourself to help strengthen your back and at the same time reduce your pain and your stress.

Biofeedback is worth considering as a way to slow down or defeat pain. Initially biofeedback is done under the guidance of a therapist, but the techniques you learn can be used later at home.

Acupressure is successfully used by many for pain relief. Closely aligned with acupuncture the main difference is the use of the thumb, fingers and hand for the pressure on the vital points, rather then the needles. It works for a lot of people. Maybe it will work for you to help reduce your sciatica pain, even if it's only for a few hours.

Reflexology seems a little bit exotic at first hearing to some people. But it really is a very simple practice that involves the application of pressure, stretches, and movement to the hands and feet with the belief that this will affect corresponding parts of the body. The practice may work by transporting signals through the peripheral nervous system into the central nervous system which are then processed in various parts of the brain. Thousands of people swear by the practice and it might just work for your sciatica pain.

Homeopathy is practically made for the self-helper. There are homeopathy professionals out there and you certainly can consult one. However there is a lot of information out there for someone who wants to learn about this on his or her own. Homeopathy formulas are generally so mild and non-toxic that they can't possibly hurt you. Take a spin around your local health food store, or check online, to see the many formulas that are available including ones that are specifically designed for pain relief and even back pain.

Watching your weight. Yes, you have no doubt heard it before, carrying around extra weight puts more of a strain on your back and losing some of those extra pounds can sometimes be all it takes to free yourself of back pain. Your lumbar spine is the end of the line for carrying the load of your upper body weight. The more weight it has to support the more things can go wrong. Your weight might not be a factor in your back pain, but it could be. The odds are you'll have a healthier, less painful back if your spine has less weight to support.

Burn more calories than you put in. Simple formula to quote, hard one to follow through on in real life. The best way to burn off fat and calories is with aerobic exercises. No, not the hard driving stepping, dancing, jumping and jolting you see on TV and in the gyms. Aerobic exercise is any workout that is done on a continuous basis for twenty minutes or more.

The best is swimming, the next best is walking, and a close third is bicycling. Walking is by far the most convenient, takes the least special equipment and can be done almost anywhere. Combine exercise with healthy eating and your bound to beat the battle of the bulge.

Don't sign up for a fancy diet. Don't buy specialty diet food. Simply read the labels and eat no more than twenty-two to thirty-eight fat grams a day if you're a woman. Men should not eat more than twenty-eight to sixty grams of fat a day.

Read the labels on prepared food. You'll be surprised how quickly you can go over those totals. Splurge every once in awhile but be ware of how many grams of fat you can rack up with just one splurge. For example a breakfast of sausage, eggs and hash browns will kick in with thirty-four grams of fat. The average fast food hamburger will nail you with from forty-five to sixty grams of fat. A three-quarter pound steak dinner with all the trimmings will set you back one hundred and sixty fat grams.

Those First Few Exercises

There is a whole chapter on exercises later in the book. But right about now as your back is getting better, is the time to start with some gentle and easy exercises. The rule is: if it hurts, don't do it.

Walking

If you're overweight and out of shape, start a walking program to go along with your regular exercise program. The walking combined with your lower intake of fat and calories will help you take off weight. The exercises will help strengthen your muscles. The combination is going to help your back to get better and when it's well help it to stay in better shape.

One of the reasons that walking is such a great exercise is because of its flexibility. It's easy to do, requires no special equipment besides a pair of decent athletic shoes, and you can do it anywhere and anytime. You can walk by yourself or with one or a dozen others. You can walk faster or slower as the mood or your time slot or your energy level indicates. You can vary your route to keep things interesting.

Walking is also a great, underrated, calorie burner. Walking at four miles an hour for fifteen minutes uses up one hundred calories. It gives your whole body a workout, your lungs, your legs, your back, and your heart. It helps to relieve the stress of everyday living and improves your mood.

Sure you can burn calories faster with running. But running on paving or black-top or even a hard packed path can give your knees and your back a series of continual jolts each time your weight comes down on one foot. Too many of these jolts can do a lot of damage.

Swimming

Swimming is an almost perfect exercise, working more of your body's muscles at the same time than almost any other aerobic workout you can do. Even better there is almost zero stress on your bones and cartilage as you burn off up to one hundred forty-five calories in fifteen minutes.

Bicycling

With biking there is relatively little equip-
ment needed: just a bike and a helmet. You can use any kind of bike that fits your price range and style, from a higher end mountain bike to the old fashioned touring bike style. It also burns a good amount of calories. Bicycling at just ten miles an hour on a level route will use up one hundred five calories in fifteen minutes.

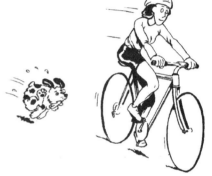

If you have lower back pain, like sciatica, biking is often a good choice because it allows you to get moving burning calories and building muscle but it doesn't cause further stress to your hurting back.

Biking also offers flexibility in your workout. You can do it outside along residential streets or in parks or special bike paths. You can also get the same results without ever leaving your house using your stationary bike.

Be sure to warm up gradually before doing any hard riding. In fact it's best to avoid any strenuous workout when you are having a flare-up of pain.

When you are still experiencing pain take it easy on the bike inside or out. Outside, don't try to work up any hills and, inside, don't put on much resistance. Go the easy route until your pain starts to subside. Try tougher rides as you get stronger. Listen to your body. It will tell you when you're ready to move on to the harder exercising.

Bicycling at ten miles an hour on a level route will use up one hundred five calories in fifteen minutes. Not bad and does more than walking.

Stress Relief

Experts say that stress can be a big contributor to back pain. Relieve your stress and you may help to relieve your back pain from sciatica or some other problem.

Stress is an emotional problem, not a physical one, but the emotions can often affect the physical in a powerful manner. To make matters worse your back pain may contribute to your stress level creating essentially a pain stress loop. This loop effect is magnified if you have a back pain or sciatica that is giving you fits for months.

Sciatica back pain can disturb your sleep at night causing extreme fatigue. It can affect your concentration on the job. If the pain is so bad you are forced to miss work this can eat away at your self-respect not to mention the stress inducing money troubles that may follow.

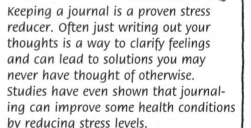

TAME THE PAIN TIP

Keeping a journal is a proven stress reducer. Often just writing out your thoughts is a way to clarify feelings and can lead to solutions you may never have thought of otherwise. Studies have even shown that journaling can improve some health conditions by reducing stress levels.

Interestingly many people don't even recognize when they are feeling stressed. Stress affects almost everyone differently. It shows up in a wide variety of emotional and physical responses. Here are some common signs of stress. See if one or more of them fit you:

- Feeling intense pressure on the job and at home
- A feeling of being overwhelmed
- Extreme impatience
- Loss of interest in usually enjoyable activities
- Muscle tension

■ Extreme nervousness

■ Withdrawing from usual activities

■ Problems with concentration

■ Low "flash point" of anger

■ Problems with sleeping

■ Trembling for no apparent reason

■ A sudden, radical change in appetite

Do any of these common stress-indicators sounds familiar to you? If so, you probably are a victim of stress, whether you are aware of it or not. This stress no doubt is aggravating your sciatica symptoms. So now the next step is to reduce your stress levels, which in turn should reduce your pain.

Try these methods:

■ Start by taking a look at your life, your life style. Try writing down a list of things that are causing stress in your life. Now look over the list and start editing out activities and conditions in your life that are not absolute musts. For those unavoidable stress-producing situations adopt the "Be Cool" attitude. Try to relax and cope with them in a gentle, easygoing way. It won't always work, but give it a try.

■ Check local mental heath centers to see if there are any classes you can take on controlling stress. Often these are given at community centers and many are free.

■ Read everything you can find on stress management. Often these books are available in your city library. Some are on tape. Also check your local bookstore for books and tapes on stress.

■ If you have high blood pressure, anxiety attacks or headaches you think are brought on by stress, talk with your doctor about it. He may have some medications that will help, and some life style changes for you to put into practice.

- You may wish to investigate special programs such as biofeedback, which can help you with your stress levels. A specialist in the biofeedback field handles these.

- Your doctor may want to refer you to a specialist, such as a psychologist, who can advise you and work with you in special techniques to manage and lower your stress level.

There is no chance that we can go into all of the ramifications of stress management here. It's a huge subject, complicated and with dozens of techniques and programs. Hundreds of books have been written on the subject.

What we want to do here is to remind you that stress plays a part in your sciatica pain, and that you need to be aware of it, and not to let it take over you life.

Stress is a factor, but the more you know about it, and anticipate it, and move to short circuit it, the better off you will be.

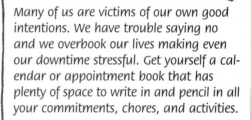

TAME THE PAIN TIP

Many of us are victims of our own good intentions. We have trouble saying no and we overbook our lives making even our downtime stressful. Get yourself a calendar or appointment book that has plenty of space to write in and pencil in all your commitments, chores, and activities.

Take a good hard look. Are your days to packed? Have your double-booked yourself and over-committed? Are you simply trying to do too much? Bow out gracefully from any commitments that have you overbooked or double-booked. Now make a commitment to yourself to keep your calendar up to date and to not overdo. Try even scheduling in downtime to relax and reduce your stress levels.

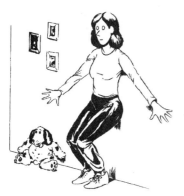

Chapter Seven:

Yes, Exercise DOES Help

So, let's say you've had a bad sciatic attack, maybe the first one, maybe not. You've seen the doctor and tried some of the self help ideas and guess what... you're getting better. Generally, little by little, the pain is starting to recede.

Now that you're getting better you probably remember that at some point your doctor mentioned that exercising would help you do better and in the long run help your back and stomach to have stronger muscles which would aid in preventing another sciatic attack.

At the time your doctor first mentioned it you probably couldn't even think about exercising. But now that the pain is receding it's time to get serious about it. The fact is if you build up your muscles through your middle, often referred to as the core muscles, you can help avoid future back problems.

Warm Up Before Exercising

You should always warm up before exercising. This is especially important for those of us with back trouble. Five minutes on a stationary bicycle or a five-minute brisk walk can get your body ready for your exercise and prevent further injuries.

For those of you who are still having considerable back pain, but still want to do an exercise program, you may want to opt for a hot shower warm up for now. The hot water warms up the muscles and gets you ready for your workout. Your goal is to be able to do some light exercise comfortably to gain three main sciatica-busting benefits.

■ Exercise can help stretch the area of your lumbar spine back to normal

■ Exercise helps your body become more flexible increasing your normal range of movement

■ Exercise helps strengthen muscles compensating for any lax ligaments that can't be tightened in your back.

Exercise During and After an Attack

Much will depend on how much you hurt, how far along you are with your recovery and what the doctor told you to do. If you're in the two-month "rehabilitation" period after an attack, you might not want to do any more exercising than a gentle walk around the house.

If you're past that stage, here are some gentle exercises and stretches you can try. **Remember, if it hurts, stop doing it!**

By this time you probably can walk around the house a little. This is a good

THE GLUTEAL-SQUEEZE

Part of maintaining a healthy back is maintaining the gluteal muscles in the buttocks. The gluteal muscles provide support for the spine during daily activities like sitting, walking, and standing. This simple gluteal-squeeze, which both strengthens the muscles in the buttocks and loosens the spine, should be incorporated into your daily routine. It's so easy to do and non-strenuous that even if you are stuck in bed the first day or so after an attack you can do it.

● Lie on your back and gently bring your knees up keeping your feet flat on the floor. If this causes any discomfort, say right after an attack, you can also leave your legs lying straight.

● Gently squeeze the muscles in our buttocks increasing the squeeze until they are as tight as you can get them and then slowly relax. Repeat this squeeze at least 50 and up to 100 times twice a day.

time to move it outside and try to walk a block. If you can do that the first day you try it, do it for a week, then perhaps try a little longer walk. Walking is one of the best exercises for the body, despite what they say about the exercise machines and gadgets on TV. If the pain lets you, keep building up your walk until you can go a considerable distance without pain. Walking is an exercise? You bet.

If you don't want to walk, you might try one of the other good exercises for post sciatic patients. One is swimming. This again can be done a little at a time, on your own schedule, increasing the length of time spent at is as you feel ready. You are building up your muscles for your whole body, including your back.

If you choose to try swimming it's best to avoid the breast stroke. This stroke requires arching the spine sharply and this can irritate your already painful sciatica area. The breast stroke is also bad for some people with specific kinds of back disease and pain. Check with your doctor to be sure. Generally, avoid the breast stroke and use one of the other resting strokes such as the side stroke.

Bicycling is another exercise that

TAME THE PAIN TIP

Water exercise is an excellent non-impact form of aerobic workout. You perform simple body movements in shallow water. It is especially helpful to those who suffer from back pain or arthritis because it supports the body, cushioning the joints and muscles, while giving you an excellent work out.

Exercising in water can be tough so don't have unrealistic expectations. Deeper water can mean the resistance to movement is as high as that with heavy free weights. Those with back problems need to be especially cautious when doing any kind of exercise including water aerobics.

If possible take a class with an instructor. Your local YMCA or gym will most likely offer classes. Talk with the instructor first and learn what level of difficulty the routines are and discuss your special needs. Adapt some of the higher resistance exercise if needed to put less stress on your back.

Working out in a heated pool gives several benefits besides the resistance factor. The warm water helps circulation and can give a high psychological boost as well. Exercises can also be done with flotation devices to help make them easier to perform.

can be good for sciatica sufferers. Again, here you'll want to take it gently and easily at first, maybe only a block or two. If getting on and off the bike gives you lots of pain, this one isn't for you.

If you feel comfortable on the bike do the usual build up of a little more each week until you are getting a good workout. As you go a little farther each time, you'll be building up your back and abdominal muscles and strengthening them, which could help you avoid another sciatic attack.

Remember if It Hurts, STOP! It's worth repeating. Rule number one for doing any type of exercise, especially after a sciatica attack, is that if it causes pain you should stop at once. There are dozens of exercises that you can try that shouldn't irritate your sensitive back.

Stretching It Out

So now your back is feeling better, but it's not a hundred percent yet. You need some in-between exercises to help you get back in shape and strengthen your back and abs. But before doing these, or any other exercises you, are going to need to do some stretching. You need to get your muscles stretched out so they won't suddenly scream and yell at you as you go down in a heap.

For most of us, over the years, some of our ligaments stretch and sag. Other parts of our body may then contract and shorten to compensate. If there are any shortened muscles in your back or along your spine, they may be contributing to the reason for your back hurt in the first place. By stretching these out they will have the chance to get back in their proper position while prepping your body for slightly more intense exercise.

Stretch #1: Static Hamstring Stretch

Your hamstring muscles begin in your buttocks and go down the back of each leg and fasten to the back of your knees. When you stretch your hamstring, you normally will also be stretching your sciatic nerve. However, if you're just recover-

ing from sciatic pain or have had several
bouts with it, you should stretch your ham-
strings statically. This one will not stretch
your sciatic nerve and will not interrupt the
healing process.

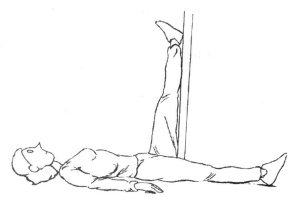

To do this stretch, lie on your back near a
doorway. Move your buttocks next to the
door jamb.

Extend your right leg through the doorway and the lift your left leg so it rests
on the door jamb. Keep your leg straight. Move your buttocks forward until all of
your leg touches the door jamb. Don't let your knee bend.

Hold the leg in position for a full minute. Relax. Then change legs and extend
the other leg against the door jamb for a full minute.

Stretch #2: The Pelvic Tilt

For this stretch lie on your back on the floor
or other hard surface. Bend your knees up to a
forty-five degree angle and keep your feet flat
on the floor. Relax the muscles of your legs and
feet.

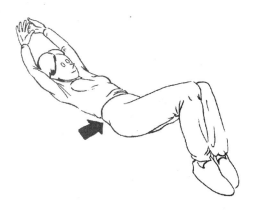

Breathe normally. Press your lower back flat
against the floor. Do this by tightening your
abdominal muscles. This will make your hip
joint roll toward your stomach. Hold this position for ten seconds and then relax. Repeat this
procedure twenty-five times.

After you are comfortable with this stretch, try extending one leg to lie flat on
the floor, all the while maintaining the pelvic tilt and with your lower back flat on
the floor. Now bend the leg upward to the original position without losing the tilt.
This is harder.

Stretch #3: Standing Pelvic Tilt

After you master the lying pelvic tilt, try this one standing up.

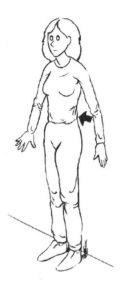

Stand and put your back against a wall with your heels about two inches from it. Lean your head against the wall and look straight ahead. Push your lower back gently toward the wall. Try to make your back as flat against the wall as you can and eliminate the hollow spot. Be sure not to hold your breath or tighten up your bottom. Press back for twenty seconds, then relax. Do this stretch twenty times.

Note: this stretch is a good one to do to relieve tension in your

Eleven Stretches You Should NEVER Do

1. From sitting position, stretching head forward and resting it on your legs or ankles. Too much stress on your lower back.

2. From a standing position, lifting one leg to the rear and pulling upward with your hand on the ankle. Creates bad spine alignment.

3. From standing position, bend and touch right toe with left hand, then reverse. Too much pressure in lower back.

4. From standing position, lay leg on tabletop and stretch upper body forward to touch leg. Too much stress on lower back.

5. From standing position, bend over and touch toes or put hands flat on the floor. Over stress on lower back.

6. From prone position, stretching upper body upward on fully extended arms and arching head and neck backwards. Neck arch puts too much stress on upper neck and spine.

7. Sitting with legs crossed in lotus position and rounded back. Too much stress on lower back.

8. Sitting with one leg extended, other one to the side and stretching torso and head forward to touch extended leg. Bad for the lower back.

9. Rolling of the head too far to the back. Overstretches the neck and upper spine.

10. Lying down, arms extended, lift legs over head and try to touch toes to floor behind head. Over stretches lower back.

11. A shoulder stand, with legs extended fully directly above shoulders. Serious pressure on upper neck bones.

back and help relieve mild back pain anytime.

Stretch #4: The Low Back Stretcher

This one should be on every-one's list. It can relax your back muscles, ease tension, wipe out pains and aches in your shoulders and do a whole lot of good.

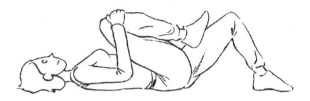

Lie on the floor with your head down. Move one leg to a forty-five degree angle with your foot on the floor. Lift the other leg up and gently pull it to your chest with both arms.

If there is pain due to a recent sciatica attack, bring your thigh as close to your chest as you can without any pain. As the pain lessens, you can try bringing your thigh closer and closer until it touches your chest. Hold it there for ten seconds and then return it to the bent knee position. Repeat this ten times on the first leg, the switch legs.

After you've stretched both legs, take a thirty second break, then lift both legs to your chest and tighten your arms. Hold for ten seconds. Do this double stretch ten times.

Stretch #5: Low Back Half Press Up Stretch/Rest Position

This one may be the single most important stretch or exercise in the book. It's the only tested and proven stretch to be done after a sciatica attack. It's an ideal flexor for the spine.

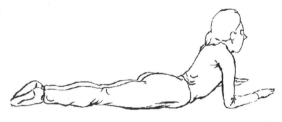

Lie on your stomach on a hard surface. Keep your hands, forearms and elbows flat on the surface. Lift your head and shoulders off the floor and look straight ahead keeping your elbows firmly on the surface. This gently arches your back.

Hold for 10 seconds and then relax. Do a series of ten to fifteen of these to help relax your back. As you get more flexible, try straightening your arms.

Back Strengthening Exercises

So, your back and legs are feeling better. Most or all of the pain of the sciatica is gone. You want something more to help keep your back in better shape so you don't run the risk of another sciatica attack. Good strengthening exercises can help. Below are a bunch that can be done without the use of weights. They use the weight of your body itself to get the job done.

If you think you're ready for work to help make your back stronger and you try some of these exercises and they hurt stop the exercise at once. The rule still is, if it hurts, don't do it.

Also a vital warning about sit-ups. Do not do full sit-ups with legs flat on the floor and coming up into a full sitting position. This causes a lot of strain on your lumbar spine area and can create or worsen lumbar problems. Don't do full sit up with your toes hooked under a couch or having someone hold them for you for the same reason.

Exercise #1: The Half Sit-Up

This exercise is done to make your abdominals stronger. These half sit-ups are a good way to tighten up and make your abdominals flatter.

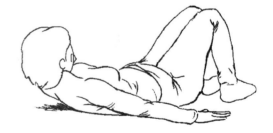

Lie on the floor with your knees bent and feet flat. Rest your arms at your sides or on your abdomen. Tuck in your chin and push your arms forward lifting your head and shoulders off the floor. Don't go too high. Hold this position for ten seconds, then return your head and shoulders to the floor.

This one will soon make your abdominals start to burn and hurt. Stop. The next time you'll be able to do more. Work up to twenty. Then if you want more, take a short break and do another set of twenty. Don't correctly these can't hurt your back and will help wonderfully well with your abdominals.

Exercise #2: Partial Leg Lift

This one will help strengthen muscles in your knees, abdomen and the front of your hip. If done correctly, they will also help you to keep your spine and pelvis stable when you move your legs, which will help you to sit and bend properly.

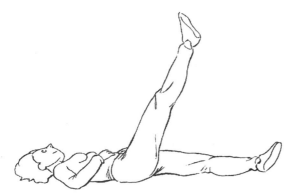

Lying flat on the floor, place hands on each side of lower abdomen. Your lower back should be lying flat on the floor. Lift one leg to a seventy-degree angle keeping your knee straight. Hold leg up for seven counts, then lower it to the floor. Don't let your trunk and pelvis move as you lift or lower your leg.

Now repeat with the other leg. Do this exercise from seven to twenty-five times, depending on your strength.

Exercise #3: Half Squat Rotation

This exercise is designed to build more strength in your legs and to help improve your balance.

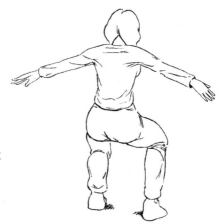

Begin standing with feet spread apart a little more than normal so they are directly under your shoulders. Do a half squat and hold it, then move slowly in a circular motion shifting your weight in a circle around your feet. At all times keep your trunk and head in a straight up position. You may want to use your arms as a counterbalance as you move around. Your legs will show strain first. Do for fifteen to twenty seconds. Stand and rest legs, then do two more repetitions.

Exercise #4: The Bridge

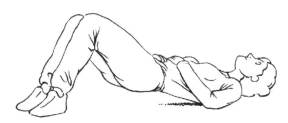

Here you can work on strengthening your buttocks, back, thighs and abdominals. With practice it will help you to stand taller, climb stairs easier, and get up from a low chair without strain.

Lie on back with knees drawn up to forty-five degree angle. Slowly tighten lower abdominals and buttocks to flatten your lower back to the floor. Now lift your pelvis off the floor an inch or two at a time until your pelvis and low back come off the floor. Tighten your buttocks as you lift. This forms a bridge between your feet and your upper back and shoulders. Hold position for five seconds as you breathe normally.

Now lower your pelvis slowly an inch at a time until you again have your lower back flat on the floor. Do this exercise from seven to fifteen times.

Exercise #5: Leg Lifts While Standing

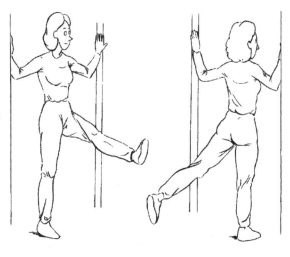

By consistently practicing this exercise you can strengthen most of the major muscles in your legs. When you maintain good head, pelvis and trunk position during the workout, you will further aid in maintaining a good posture. This one can also help with your balance and coordination.

Always use a desk or doorway for balance when doing these exercises and maintain good posture throughout.

Hold on to a doorway with both hands, keeping your head and trunk directly over your hips as you lift one straight leg forward as high as you can without moving your torso. Go only as high as you can comfortably. Hold the leg at height for eight seconds, and then slowly lower it. Repeat ten to twenty times with each leg.

Now do much the same thing lifting the leg to the back. Lift as high as possible without changing your torso or head position and hold for eight seconds. Then lower leg slowly. Repeat with each leg, both forward lifts and backward lifts, for ten to twenty times.

Exercise #6: Abdominal Leg Extensions

Helping to strengthen your abdominal muscles is an important part in healing sciatica problems as well as other back hurts. Your abdominal muscles are what support your spine and pelvis from both sides and the front. Since these muscles are so active in supporting the spine, they must be worked smoothly, with no straining, jerking or high-speed repetitions. This is one of a number of abdominal exercises you can do.

Start by lying on your back with both knees in bent up position. Slowly push out your right leg until it is straight and six inches off the 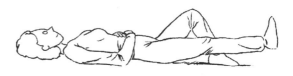 floor. Keep your back and abdomen straight and back flat on floor. Hold leg off floor three to five seconds, then pull it back slowly bending your knee and placing foot on floor in bent knee position. This is a hard one. Do three to five times on one leg, then switch to the other leg.

When you can hold each leg off the floor for ten to fifteen seconds for ten reps, try the same thing only with both legs at the same time. This one is for advanced exercisers only.

Exercise #7: Hand And Foot Extensions

You've probably never heard of your extensor muscles. They run along your back in your buttocks, thighs shoulders and neck. These are the muscles that hold your spine stable and help you maintain your balance. This hand and foot extension exercise will help strengthen these muscles and in turn help keep your spine straight and strong.

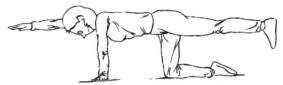

Get on the floor on your hands and knees, keeping your back straight and your head and neck in line with your back. Shift your weight to your right knee, lift your left leg and fully extend it backwards keeping it level with the floor. At the same time shift your weight to your left hand and fully extend your right arm forward keeping it parallel with the floor. Hold the position for three to seven seconds.

Return both hand and foot to the floor. Repeat this action seven to twelve times on each side.

Exercise #8: Side Leg Lifts

This exercise is designed to build up the muscles that give stability to your lower back, hips and pelvis. Done consistently they can help you to maintain good posture putting less strain on your back.

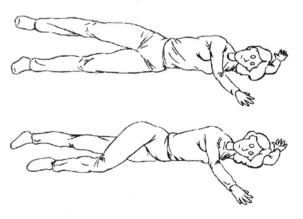

Lie on the side with your head on a pillow or on your bent arm. Your top arm should be extended in front of you for balance so you won't roll forward. Your legs rest on top of each other. Now rotate your top leg upward, keeping your knee straight to about eighteen inches off the floor. Hold that position for three to seven seconds, and then slowly return it to its original position. Repeat this twelve to twenty times.

Now move your top leg forward with bent knee and put it on the floor freeing the bottom leg. Lift the bottom leg off the floor as far as comfortable and hold for three to seven seconds then slowly return it to the floor. Repeat this twelve to twenty times.

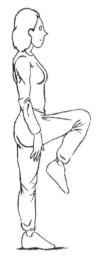

Exercise #9: Leg Lift Balance

This simple exercise will help to train your abdominal and back muscles to lengthen and support your spine as well as help with your basic balance.

Stand with your feet about a foot apart. Stand tall as you tighten your lower abdominal muscles. As you keep them tight, lift one knee waist high and hold it there for five seconds. Use your hands at first if you need to, to maintain your balance.

After five seconds, lower leg and lift the other one for five seconds. Do each leg ten times alternating.

Exercise #10: Side Bends

This is another easy one that can help limber up your back and at the same time strengthens your side torso muscles. It's a good one to do after an attack when you have been unable to do your routine for a while to help you get back to moving.

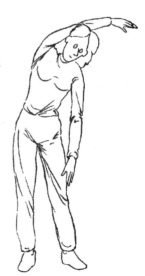

Stand with your feet about eighteen inches apart. Reach your right arm down toward your knee and at the same time lift your left arm over your head and bend it as far to the right as you can. Bend only as far as is comfortable and never bounce as this can cause further injury and pain. Return left arm to your side and do the same thing on your left side stretching with your right arm over your head.

Repeat on each side from five to ten times.

Exercise #11: Spine Rotations

This exercise is designed to limber up your spine. Spinal rotation is required in many daily activities and this is a good way to keep your spine ready for a work or play.

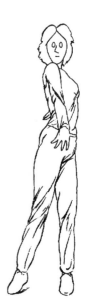

Stand with your feet about sixteen inches apart, hold arms away from body to side at about a forty-five degree angle. Rotate your torso and head to the left as if looking back over your shoulder. As you do this let your right heel come off the floor. Tighten your lower abdominals to support your lower back. This twisting motion will help your whole spine to do a gentle rotation. Hold this position for five seconds, return to the start.

Now do the same maneuver twisting to the right as if looking over your right shoulder. Again, hold for five seconds. Repeat this from five to ten times on each side.

Exercise #12: The Resting Clam

If your lower back starts to feel tired or tight, this is a good exercise to help loosen it up and to rest.

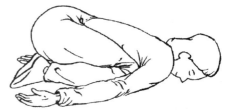

Kneel on the floor and then gently bend forward with your chest against your thighs lowering your head to the floor and extending your arms back along your legs (see illustration on the right).

Do this one very slowly. It will come easier with practice. When you can do the position fully, maintain it for fifteen to thirty seconds, then lift up and relax. Repeat for three to five times depending on how you feel.

Exercise #13: Leg Thruster

Start by lying on your back with both knees pulled to your chest. Then hold left knee and extend right leg to ninety-degree vertical position keeping your foot flat on top. (Don't point your toe upward.)Hold this position for five to ten seconds until you feel a stretch in the back of your leg. Return right leg to chest.

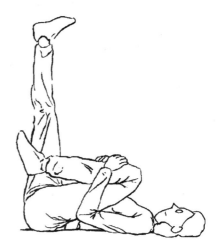

Now hold your right leg and extend your left leg upward as you did the right one and hold for five to ten seconds. Then return it to your chest.

Repeat this exercise on both sides from five to ten times.

Exercise #14: Gentle Abs Workout

Here is a simple abdominal exercise that can be increased in intensity as you build your abs.

Sit on the floor with your knees bent at a forty-five degree angle, your torso is held erect and your arms folded and held away from your chest almost at shoulder height.

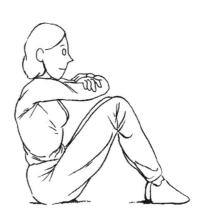

Now, lean your torso backward a little at a time until you feel your abdominals tightening. Hold this position for five to fifteen seconds while continuing to sit tall. Look straight ahead during this lean. Then return to the starting position. Repeat this exercise from five to ten times. As you build up your abdominal muscles you can increase the angle of the lean to increase the intensity.

Exercise #15: Holding Up The Wall

With this exercise you are strengthening both your torso and legs. The lower you slide down along the wall the more the movement will work your legs. You can adjust the depth of the movement to adjust the intensity of the workout. Easy does it here.

Stand with your back against a wall and your arms at your sides. Slowly slide down the wall for about two feet and then slide back up. The lower you slide down, the more pressure you'll put on your legs. Work your abs on the top side of the wall. If you slide down too far, and can't get back up, gently go down to your knees, get up and try it again.

Repeat five of the easier slides.

Exercise #16: Chair Bend Down

For a general back stretch that won't kill you, try this gentle chair bend. Work both sides and hold as long as you feel comfortable.

Sit on a chair for this one and bend forward so your chest is touching your knees. Extend both arms and lean to the right so you can put your clasped hands outside your right foot. Hold five seconds. Return to upright position. Now bend forward and lean to the left and put clasped hands outside your left foot. Repeat on each side from five to ten times.

Exercise #17: The Sidewinder Slide

The sidewinder will help work your abs and your leg muscles as well. Remember to slide, not lift your leg on this one.

Lie on your left side with knees and hips slightly bent. Cushion your head on your folded arm. Now slide your right leg upward until you can bring it as close to your chest as possible. Hold in that position for five seconds and slide it back down to the starting position. Repeat five times.

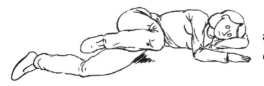 Then roll over on your right side and slide the left leg the same as you did the right one, repeating five times.

Your Exercise Plan

You of course aren't going to want to do all of these exercises every single day. Try them and pick out the ones that seem to help you the most. Switch them around for variety.

Remember to not overdo the exercising, especially when you start out. Also don't forget the cardinal rule in exercising to help your back: If it hurts, don't do it!

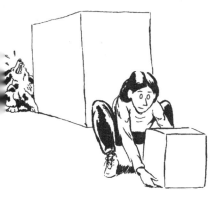

Sitting, Standing, Bending Tips

Let's just admit it at the outset: Most of us don't know a thing about good posture. We are basically clueless when it comes to what good sitting or standing posture actually is. We have no idea how to sit at a desk properly, use a keyboard the right way, or spend time at a work table without throwing our backs out of kilter. But not knowing these things has led no doubt to lots of pain filled hours, causing or aggravating your sciatica condition.

Good posture isn't all that hard, most of us are just too sloppy or unconcerned about it to care—that is until our backs give us a mighty good reason for paying attention.

Many doctors and back specialists tell us that bad posture and work habits contribute more than we know to back problems, even if they don't show up for years down the line. That's why I am going to go into quite a bit of detail in this chapter.

By making good posture a habit, you just might be able to avoid another painful sciatic attack, or some other back problem that can be caused or seriously aggravated by bad posture and bad sitting, standing, reaching and lifting habits.

Poor Sitting Habits

Most of the experts agree that just sitting in a chair or on a couch is one of the most stressful positions you can get into in relation to your low back and neck. Millions of people spend most of their day sitting down at a desk or computer terminal during their working day. Millions more spend a lot of time in arm chairs and kitchen chairs during the day at home.

Crossing Your Legs

When you cross your legs while sitting, you tip your pelvis to one side and this produces a curve in your spine. Usually this curve is temporary and will go away when you stand or move to a new position. The best way to counteract this sideways curve is to alternate your leg positions. Cross your right leg over your left the first time, then a short time later reverse the cross. This reverses the spinal curve and negates any long-term problem.

Crossing your legs in general will not cause you trouble unless you consistently cross your legs in the same manner, never shifting legs or position. Another tip is to push your pelvis firmly against the chair's back before you cross your legs. This will give you a more stable platform.

Stressful Sitting

Avoiding sitting in any position that causes you to have tightened muscles in your back or your neck just to maintain the position. Don't, for example, lean forward in your car when driving, stressing the muscles in your back. Or try not to tense up the muscles in your shoulders and back when you are stuck at your desk for hours pulling together that final report or answering e-mails. Instead push your hips against the back of a firm chair, lean back, relax and let the chair hold you in a good sitting position.

Sitting In The Same Place Too Long

In sales training there is an axiom: The mind can absorb only as much as the seat of the pants can stand. The idea was that people in meetings for over 50 minutes should be given a "seventh inning break" by standing and talking or just looking around.

We humans are not designed to sit in one position for hours at a time. Sitting is much more stressful on the spine than standing. Even if you are in a good sitting position, it's good to give the body a break and get up and move about or change your sitting position. Cross your legs the other way, move to a different chair, do some work that requires you to be standing for a time. Work out a variety of sitting positions to keep your body in better tune.

Slumped Over Sitting

When you sit slumped over or slouch in your chair your back is rounded, your tailbone tends to roll under your hips and your head is thrust forward instead of being in line with your spine.

This unnatural curve is a very stressful position for your back. If you sit this way for any length of time on a regular basis your spine can develop strange curves and your head and neck can give you a lot of problems.

This position can also increase compression and over stretching of the pelvis and lower back. Sitting this way is often the culprit in much of the low back, neck pain, and even headaches that patients feel. It also can mean problems in breathing since the diaphragm can't work correctly and your ribs don't have room to expand as they normally do.

A sofa or chair that is too soft with a poor back support can cause this back-stressing position. The best solution is to avoid this type of seating.

Good Sitting Habits

If you have to sit down for long periods for work or other reasons you should make it your business to learn a variety of ways to sit comfortably and with good posture.

The basic building block for good sitting posture is to learn to recognize where your pelvis is in relation to your chair. Most people sit down in a chair about in the middle of the seat and then slump forward either not making any contact at all with the back of the chair or lean backwards from this position causing the spine to not be aligned.

TAME THE PAIN TIP

Okay, you've been sitting there an hour, you still have a pile of work to do and can't go for a ten-minute walk. What do you do? Some body movements can help you relax and still let you keep working. Try these:

- Rocking your pelvis. Rock your pelvis and low back forward and up using the chair arms for support. Your tailbone should lift off the seat and your low back will arch forward. Hold the position for three to five seconds and repeat it four times. Then get back to work.

- If you do a lot of reading at a desk, try using a slant board that will lift the material three to six inches off your desk and make it easier to read. This will help eliminate a head down position that can be murder on your neck and spine.

- After sitting a long time, try doing your reading or writing job at a makeshift stand up desk. Sometimes a file cabinet is the right height. Twenty minutes at your make shift standing desk and you'll be ready to sit again.

- Try temporarily propping up your head with your elbow on your desk and your palm under your chin. You can still write and read, but now the muscles around your neck have support and can relax for a bit while your head still stays upright.

To master good sitting posture once seated you should move your pelvis to the rear so it contacts the back of the chair. To do this put your hands on the arms of the chair and lean forward lifting yourself up a few inches while at the same time shifting your pelvis backward until you are positioned at the back of the seat. Now lean backward allowing your upper back to make contact with the chair as well and you have a perfect sitting position. Your head, neck and spine are all in an arrow straight alignment.

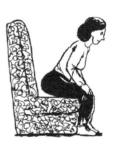 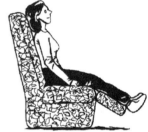

If you have a reclining seat in your car on the passenger's side, it's an ideal way to relax while maintaining good posture. Push your pelvis towards the front part of the seat, then lean back with your legs stretched forward in a fairly straight line. This should end up with your head, neck and spine all in alignment.

If you are sitting in a chair and

need to do work at a table or desk or you are eating you are going to need to lean forward in your chair. You can do this while maintaining good posture. The key is again positioning your pelvis against the back of the chair but then leaning forward keeping your head, neck and back in alignment.

You might also try moving to the front edge of your chair with your pelvis. Then leaning forward again keeping your head, neck and spine in a straight line.

Most of us are so used to sitting correctly that this may at first feel strange and you may find yourself reverting to your normal slump. Just readjust until you are in a straight line again. Eventually it will become second nature and trust me, your back will thank you for it.

Lumbar Supports

Lumbar supports are small pillow-like devices that are used to help support your lower back by maintaining the natural curve. They come in various sizes and shapes so you might need to experiment to find one that fits you just right. You might want to test with a rolled up magazine or a towel to get an idea of what size support you need.

Once you have purchased your support you are going to want to find the perfect position for you. Sit correctly in your chair (pelvis pushed to back of chair) and place the support in the curve of your back then sit back and check how it feels.

Move the support up or down until you find the spot that give you the most support. Once you find the right spot, you may wish to tie or tape the support against the back of your chair. That way it won't slip or fall out and it will be there every time you sit down.

Poor Standing Habits

A good standing position is one that supports the body in a perfectly balanced stance while using relatively little muscle energy to do it. When you look at a standing figure from the side, there should be a straight line from the ear, down through the body, through the middle of the leg and to the foot. No forward thrust of the chest or the buttocks pushed out to the rear. Sounds fairly simple, but the doing is always tougher than the saying. Fact is few of us have good posture when we stand.

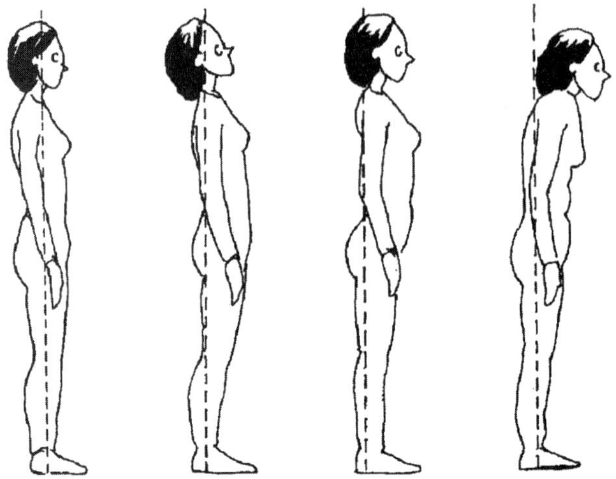

Figure 8:
Good standing posture means that your head neck spine and legs should all be in arrow-straight alignment like the first figure. The other three figures represent common poor standing-posture habits.

Correct standing puts less pressure on your spine than sitting down or a variety of other movements. Try to keep it that way with good posture.

Standing tall is a term many physical therapists use to urge their patients to pull in their stomachs, pull in their buttocks and get a more straight-line posture. Any time you find yourself slipping remind yourself to stand tall.

The Leaning Crane Stand

Some people have a forward leaning standing posture. This puts a lot of strain on your body. With a leaning forward stance your knees are pushed backwards and locked into place. This tends to tip the pelvic and low back area to forward increasing the arch in your back. This position also may push down the chest bringing the head and neck into a forward and dropped down position.

The leaning crane is extremely stressful on body muscles Since it makes you feel like you're going to fall forward your body muscles compensate by pulling back to keep you standing.

If you're guilty of this bad posture habit it's time to change it. First unlock your knees, allowing them to move forward so they bend slightly and so they are directly above your ankles. Your new knee position will automatically help you level your pelvis so it is better aligned over your legs. Now taking a deep breath lift your chest so it is aligned over your pelvis. Lift your head and straighten your neck so you have a straight line from your ear, down your spine, through your pelvis and down your leg.

This new corrected posture will take a lot of strain off your lower back and at the same time reduce muscle use and tension.

The Slump Stand

Some people stand with have a rounded back and their head thrust forward. The slump stander tilts his pelvis outward and bends his knees to far throwing the body out of alignment.

> ## TAME THE PAIN TIP
>
> *If you have a job that forces you to stand the majority of the time such as washing dishes or working at a bench, it's a good idea to have a foot stool nearby so you can lift one foot on the stool. After a few minutes shift sides resting your other foot on the stool. Also if it's a one handed job, leaning on one arm from time to time can also help to reduce the strain on your spine.*
>
> *If you are in a situation that is going to cause you to stand for a long period of time, simply leaning back against a wall or counter from time to time will help support your body and assist with decompressing your spine.*
>
> *You also can try a simple sway. Shift your weight slightly from one foot to the other or rock forward onto your toes and then back to your heels. This will help to reduce some of the strain on your back from standing.*

To correct a slump-standing posture unlock your knees and bring them back to a normal position (slightly bent). Pull back your shoulders straighten your neck and head. As you do this you chest will come up and your rounded back will be gone. Imagine a straight line running down your side from head to ankle and your body should be aligned with that line.

Lifting and Bending

Simply bending the wrong way or lifting the wrong way can cause a bout of back pain and could trigger your sciatica. There are definite right and wrong ways to bend and lift. Below I have listed some right ways to do the job.

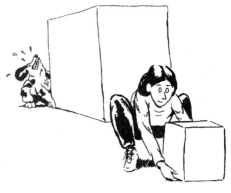

❶ To lift something off the floor, squat in front of it with your knees wide, keeping your back straight, pick up the item, and then using your legs, come upright with the pressure of the rise on your legs. Keep your back straight at all times. You may squat either with your feet flat on the floor, or on your toes, whichever way is best for you.

❷ When bending down or squatting, keep your feet wider apart than your shoulders to give yourself a good working foundation.

❸ If you're leaning forward to do a task, like taking clothes out of a front load dryer, lean one hand or arm on the top of the dryer and extend one leg behind you to help keep your spine straight as you work.

❹ If carrying suitcases or packages, balance your load on each side for equal stressing. If this is not possible, change the hand carrying the load fairly frequently to balance out the stress.

❺ When reaching or lifting something over your head, keep your body in alignment to reduce the strain. Use a step stool for overhead lifting if possible.

❻ When picking something up from the floor, do the baseball squat with knees bent and arms resting on your knees. Go down easily and pick up the light object, then push off knees with your hands to stand.

❼ Do the crane bend to pick up something near a table or chair. Rest one hand on the chair, extend one leg out behind you keeping your spine and back straight, bend down and pick up the item, then push up with your hand and return the stretched leg to a standing position.

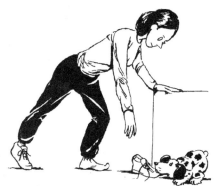

❽ The half kneeling bend is good for working on or near the floor. Bend down with one knee on the floor, the other knee bent. Especially good if your back still hurts. Keep your back perfectly straight during this move and there should be no pain.

❾ Squatting is not a good idea if you are working on the floor, such as picking up a lot of spilled items, or scrubbing or waxing the floor by hand. Instead of squatting, get down on all fours and then use one hand to do the work with the other hand helping to brace your body. This is the easiest on your back. Even sitting down and bending over to do work on the floor will excessively strain your back.

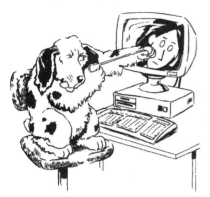

Chapter Nine:

Sciatica in the Workplace

How your physical work environment is set up as well as your work habits themselves can have an effect on your sciatica. By making a few simple changes to your work space and changing a few of your work habits that are detrimental to your back health you might be able to avoid countless hours of future sciatica pain.

Your Work Station

First let's look at a typical computer work station. Millions of people these days spend most of the day in front of a computer. Many of these workers experience back problems because things are not set up to be ergonomically correct.

A back problem at a poorly designed work station can certainly be a factor in a sciatica attack. Let's take a closer look at a computer work space and see what needs to be done.

Your Chair

The first factor to check is your work chair. A chair that is adjusted correctly for your height and weight can improve your circulation and help prevent backaches and fatigue.

Sit in your work chair and move your hips against the back, then straighten up into your usual work position. Are you comfortable? Can you reach your keyboard and other items that you need in your working day? Does the backrest fit snugly against your back? If it does not, you should adjust the backrest until your lower back is supported fully.

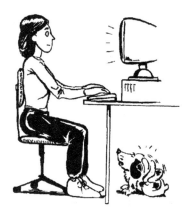

If your chair does not have an adjustable back rest, try to get one that does. If you can't, you may need to use a small pillow or rolled up towel against the back of the chair to help support your back properly.

Next you need to check to see if your chair is adjusted to the right height for you. A chair at the right height can prevent cramping and stiffness in your legs as well as relieve stress and tension in your shoulders, neck, and back.

Sit in your usual manner in your chair and place your fingers on the home keys of your keyboard. Your forearms should be parallel to the floor. If they are not, lower or raise your chair to a level that allows your arms to be level.

Now check your foot positions. Move your feet forward until your knees are at a ninety degree angle or slightly more. Your feet should be flat on the floor and about six inches of room between your stomach and they edge of the keyboard. You should also have three inches or so of room between your legs and the bottom of the keyboard platform if your desk has one.

Your Screen Height

Your whole work area should be arranged so you can reach everything and use your desk equipment without any strain on your back, neck, or shoulders.

Start by checking the height of your computer monitor. When you are seated in your properly adjusted chair, the top border of your screen should be level with your line of sight when you look straight ahead.

If the screen is too low, raise it with a magazine or telephone book or a block of wood under it exactly the right size. There are also screen platforms you can buy at any office supply store. If it is too high, you may have trouble lowering it. This is because many screens sit on top of the computer or on an electrical union box and electrical surge protector. In this case you might need to lift your keyboard and raise your chair height to compensate. At all costs get your screen at the right height.

Your Screen Distance

Now take a look at the distance your eyes are from the screen. This may depend on your eyesight and the focal length of your glasses or your contacts. Some people get special glasses that have the exact focal length needed for the way the operator likes to sit at the computer. This can be anywhere from eighteen to thirty inches. An adjustment is easy to make here, simply move the monitor and screen forward or backward until it is at the right distance for your eyes and your lenses.

Another important item for the computer work station is the placement and height of your document holder you will be working from. Be sure it is as high as the screen and as close to the screen as possible. This prevents moving your head and neck up and down to pick up copy from the bottom of a page eight inches below the bottom of the screen.

Your Keyboard Placement

We talked about the keyboard before in relation to your arms. Your forearms should be level with the floor when you're working. This takes into account that your wrists are also straight, and extension from your arms that are also straight.

Some keyboards have adjustments for height on the back of them. Adjust as needed. Some can be raised so they are slightly slanted. Many typists like this factor and use it. More keyboards being made now have a wrist rest built into them. This gives the lower part of your hand a convenient place to rest when not actually working to help reduce wrist strain.

Some of the new keyboards are split down the middle and set at a gentle angle with the keys angled backward away from the operator. These are said to be ergonomically easier on the worker. Try one to see if it works better for you. They do take a little getting used to, but many people love them.

Workplace Lighting

Be sure there is no glare on your screen from either inside or outside light. If there is a window in your room, place your computer screen at an angle that will not allow for glare that can interfere with easy reading.

If there is overhead lighting or a desk lamp, be sure that they don't glare off your screen. Adjust them so they are parallel or just behind your screen. Never let a desk lamp shine directly on the screen.

Try a Mini-Break

Working at a computer all day can be tiring. Give yourself a two minute mini-break at least every hour or so. One easy mini-break idea is to lean on your elbows on your desk. Cover your eyes with your cupped hands shutting out all light. Rest in the dark for a minute or so, then slowly remove your hands.

If your shoulders start cramping or hurting, try this. Raise your hands beside your head and then squeeze your shoulder blades towards each other. You'll feel the pull. Hold for five seconds. Repeat three to five times. Another good one is to shrug your shoulders up towards your ears as high as you can. You might hear some joints popping. That's good. Repeat this shrugging motion three times, then relax.

Another mini-break idea is to sit in your chair and drop your arms outside of the armrests. Now shake your hands or spin them for a few seconds. Stop and relax. Repeat three times.

For really bad cramping shoulders while working at a desk or computer, lie on the floor and pull one leg to your chest and hold it for ten seconds. Then do the other leg. After five reps on each side, pull both legs up and hold them for five seconds. You might want to do this in a private room, but the relaxing effect on your shoulders is remarkable.

Heavy Labor Work Situations

If you're a laborer, or must do some type of heavy work, much of the day it's really important to learn how to get the work done without hurting your back. A few suggestions:

- If something heavy has to be lifted, enlist the help of someone else to get the job done.

- Usually it's better to push a heavy object rather than try to pull it. Simple mechanics.

- If you do heavy lifting work you should try using a support belt. In fact some states now require them for certain types of jobs. While not a cure all, they can help support vital areas of your back under stressful lifting situations. But remember to still maintain good lifting practices.

- Know your limitations. If a job is too hard for you, don't be afraid to ask for help or to be reassigned. Many firms are well aware of back problems, and the cost of such injuries on their workmen's compensation insurance rates. Management will probably work with you.

- Don't do any lifting or pushing that you think might bring on a sciatic attack.

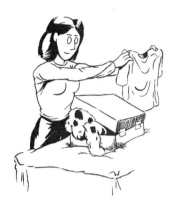

Chapter Ten:

Travel, Sleep, and Chores

Having a sciatica problem can really interfere with your daily life activities. Things that you once took for granted like traveling to see friends, getting a good night's sleep, taking the dog for a walk, or being intimate with your spouse can present real challenges when you are in pain. However making some relatively simple adjustments to your routines can make a world of difference in your quality of life.

Travel Tips

Just because you have a bad back this is no reason for you to stop enjoying life and this means you'll want to do some traveling. Following are some ideas and tips for making getting ready for travel, the trip, and the homecoming much more pleasant and a lot easier on your hurting back.

Packing Up, Getting Started

- First check out the weather at your destination, and then pack light with the proper clothing. Miami or San Diego in the summer don't require a parka and mukluks. But you'll need them if you go to Nome in December. The point is you should pack exactly what you'll need and ONLY what you need. Three out of four travelers end up packing twice the clothes they will need. Cut down your wardrobe to the minimum making your suitcase as light as possible.

■ Use the smallest suitcase that will hold what you need. If possible, get a suitcase with wheels and fold up handles for your travel. They are much simpler to move around an airport or hotel lobby and they take the strain off of your back.

■ Pack your suitcase on a bed. It's much better than bending over to the floor. Remember to take along emergency gear such as a heating pad and cold packs that can be frozen—just in case you need them.

■ Use extreme caution loading and unloading luggage into and out of your car trunk. Avoid bending forward and lifting the luggage with no support. The best idea is to pay a red cap or porter to unload your trunk and get your luggage to a check in window or curbside check station if flying.

■ If no manpower is available, use a rental or free luggage cart available in most airports and train stations to transport your bags from the curb to the check-in area.

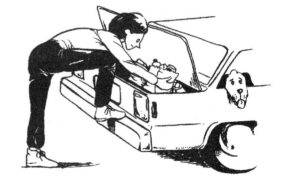

■ If you must unload luggage from your trunk. Put one foot on the bumper of the car. This will help support your back during the lift.

■ If you do strain your back with luggage or from stress, try to get an ice pack on the affected area as soon as possible. Many airports have first aid stations that can help you. Stretching out and resting while using the ice is best.

■ Wear durable, safe walking shoes for travel. Fashion is not a factor here. Many well-dressed people wear athletic shoes for traveling for their comfort and the shoe's strength and no slip qualities. Forget high-heeled shoes or those with flimsy sides or mushy soles.

■ Use the half kneeling position to pick up a heavy bag. Remember to keep changing hands if you have only one bag and must move it any great distance.

■ Traveling by train, plane or car is going to mean a lot of sitting. Use the various sitting positions we talked about before to stay comfortable. On a plane ask for two pillows to use for back and neck support. There are usually lots of pillows available. If you're on a train or in your car, bring along a favorite pillow or two for the same use.

■ Take a break. When you're driving a car or truck, be sure to stop for five minutes every hour for a break. Walk around your car, take a brisk trot a block away and back. Rest your eyes by closing them and leaning against your car for two minutes.

■ On a plane take a stand up break, walking to the back of the plane or to the bathroom. Just make sure you don't get run over by the flight attendant's beverage cart in the aisle.

■ In a car, as a passenger, lean the seat back and stretch out with your hands high over your head. Push your legs as far forward as possible and stretch as tall as you can. This can relieve a lot of pressure on your spine.

Sleeping With A Hurting Back

A lot of people with sciatica learn to dread going to bed at night because they know it's going to mean another night of increased back pain and little, if any, sleep. They know from experience that they face hours of turning and tossing and staring at the clock that seems to be running at about half its normal speed.

Let's take a look at what could be part of the problem: the foundation. What kind of a mattress do you have? Generally speaking, the experts say that a firm mattress is best for those of us with hurting backs. Why? A firm surface will tend to keep your spine from flexing as it does when your body sags into a soft mattress. That flexing can cause you pain and anguish and not allow you a whole lot of sleep.

To the basics: Find out if a firm mattress is best for your back. Take six or eight thick blankets and lay them on the floor and sleep on them for a night or two. How did it go? Did your back feel better there than on the mattress you're now using? If it did, a harder mattress is probably needed.

You can try firming up your existing bed by putting a 3/8 inch thick piece of plywood between your mattress and your box springs. One nice thing about this is that on a queen or king sized bed, this board can go on your side and not bother your spouse. The board will give you a much firmer feel to the mattress without the expense of buying a new one.

Give this a try for a week or so and see if it makes any difference. If it doesn't, your next move should be to go to a store and lie down on a variety of harder mattresses. Take some extra time with this task lying on the one you think might be your best choice for a half hour or more before making your final decision.

These days you can also choose from a variety of specialty beds like electric hospital-like beds for home use, air inflating mattresses, and memory foam mattresses. Give them all a try and see which one works best for you. This is an investment in sleeping and living pain free, so you need to be willing to invest in the right one for you.

Pre-bed Prepping

If you've been working hard all day and are still tense and tight at bedtime you might want to try some gentle stretching to relax your body and to wind down. Some simple hands over the head stretches, or some side bends and "shaking out" your hands and legs will usually be enough. Don't do any intense exercising before bed. This will elevate your heart rate and may interfere with your getting to sleep.

Time for Bed

Getting the most out of your sleep starts before you ever climb into bed. The first step is to develop a real routine you can stick to. You need to commit to going to bed at the same time every night and getting up the same time every morning. This helps program your brain and body to be ready for sleep at a certain time and to wake up at a certain time.

Next it's time to think about what position you are in when you getting ready for sleep. Most of us have a preferred sleep position that we twist into as soon as our head hits the pillow. But it may be advisable to actually have two. The first for the wind down period and the second for actual sleeping. For example you might lie on your back when you first get to bed, then after ten or fifteen minutes of relaxing you turn on your side and tuck one arm under your pillow and drop off to sleep.

Now, you're relaxed, you've had your ten minutes of "resting position" in bed, and you're ready for sleep. What's the best position for your bad back?

Most experts and back pain sufferers concur that unsupported stomach lying is hard on the back and can aggravate any kind of back pain. The key word here is "unsupported". A pillow or two often can turn a bad sleeping position into an ideal one. With the right pillows no position is really off limits.

Find the best pillow for you. If it's under your head when you lie on your back, it should be full enough so your head can rest in a position that allows a straight between head, neck and spine. Your head shouldn't fall backward or be propped too high. Either one will put a strain on your neck and spine. When lying on your back it is also a good idea to put pillows under your lower thighs and legs as well.

Now, most of us do a lot of turning while we're asleep, so how can you use a pillow when you might be on your side a half hour after you get to sleep and then on your stomach an hour later? It's a problem. Usually the pillows work best to help you get to sleep. After that unless the position is too extreme, it probably won't wake you up even when it's hurting your back a little.

One easy idea is to try a lumbar roll around your waist. This will help fill in the void when you lie down. Lumbar rolls are sold in stores, or you can make one yourself:

Take a bath towel and fold it in half lengthwise. Then roll it tightly from the side so you have a roll about three feet long. Adjust the length so it will fit snugly around your waist. It could be two to three inches thick. Now fasten it securely with safety pins so it won't slide around as you change positions at night. Try it for a night or two and see if it helps your hurting back.

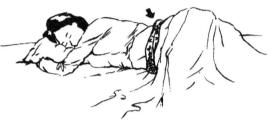

Household and Yard Work

Now for some tips for taking care of your sciatic back when you do ordinary jobs around your house, yard and garden. Many of these regular activities require a lot of lifting, bending and make repetitive movements. So the key is going to be to find ways to do these things you have done for years that will help you to avoid aggravating your back.

Gardening

You have a garden. It needs planting. The onion seedlings are waiting for you, all 120 of them in that small pack. Now how do you get those seedlings planted without killing your back?

Don't stoop over to do the job. Get a cushion or drop cloth to kneel on, then reach forward with your back straight and dig your furrow and lay the onions in. Still keeping your back straight so you won't put any undue strain on your spine. Fill in the small furrow. It's probably only a tiny adjustment from the way you used to do it, but it can really make a difference.

You can also try kneeling on one knee keeping the other foot on the ground, knee bent at your chest. You can even lean on your upper thigh for more support. Now plant as before.

A third option is to kneel down with one leg behind you and sit back on that leg keeping your other one bent so your knee is ready for resting on as you lean forward and do your planting.

Avoid sitting down and reaching forward to do your gardening. It usually doesn't work very well from a space and reach standpoint, and it is often straining on your back.

Raking Leaves

If you rake up your leaves in the fall, try doing it this way. Set your feet two feet apart and keep your whole body lined up in front. Now reach your rake out to your left or right and rake directly in front of your feet. As that area is cleaned, step forward and take another swath. This keeps your body from bending and twisting and gets the yard cleaned quicker.

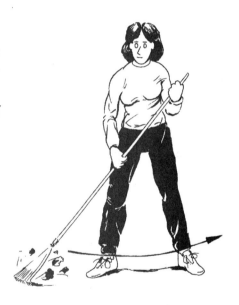

Don't stand with your feet close together and rake at your side. This will end up with you doing a lot of unnatural twisting putting pressure on all the wrong points.

Painting

Painting can be a disaster for your back, unless you do it right. Reaching high and standing on tip toes to reach that one last spot can put a lot of stress on your back and neck.

Instead use a stepladder, never going above the third step from the top so you have a place for your knees to lean against. Now, reach directly in front of you and no higher than your head and paint. This will keep your neck from cranking backward and will assure that your back remains straight so there is no undue strain on your vertebrae.

Try learning to paint with both hands if you use a brush. It may sound like a funny idea at first but it will help you to balance out the stretch of the arms and back muscles. Plus you will get the job done quicker.

Be careful or your neck may start causing you problems as you keep looking upward. If you need a taller ladder, borrow one from a neighbor or buy a 20-foot extension ladder for those high places. A longer ladder will help save your back and your neck.

Mowing the Lawn

The best way to prevent back pain from mowing the lawn is to hire a neighborhood kid to do the job. If that is not an option then try these tips. If you are using a gas engine mower the vibrations can actually irritate your back. Try wearing gloves to do the job. They will deaden some of the vibrations before they can reach your back. Wrapping the mower handles with foam rubber will help even more.

Always try to keep your back straight, arms extended and straight, and walk upright when pushing a lawn mower. Be careful not to arch your back or slip into a swayback position. Concentrate on keeping your hips in and your back straight and your eyes looking straight ahead.

Shoveling Snow

If you live in one of the cold weather states, shoveling snow comes as one of the undeniable privileges of home ownership. Again hiring the kid next door is your best bet here. Or wait a day for the sun to start to do the job. Or even better to finish it.

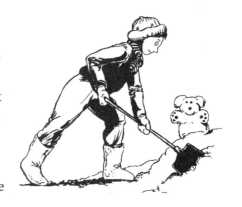

But if this is not an option you need to be sure to take all the precautions available because this particular activity can put a real hurting on your back. Shoveling snow, dirt, or gravel is one of the worst things you can do for your back. It puts a tremendous strain on it.

If you must shovel keep these things in mind.

Avoid using a huge grain shovel. A smaller shovel is often the better choice.

Your first challenge is to reach the snow without causing a strain. Avoid standing flat footed and bending over. Instead use the one foot forward, one foot back position so you can bend your front leg at the knee and lower yourself to get the shovel down to the ground. This will keep your back straight, your head up, and all in a near alignment with your trailing leg.

Fill the shovel with a reasonable amount of snow and partially lift the load by straightening out your front leg. This little trick will divert a lot of the strain of lifting away from your arms and back.

Vacuuming

Vacuuming doesn't have to be a disaster for your back, even a hurting sciatic back. Don't bend your back and lean forward as if you're in a motorcycle race. Your back will end up in pain by the time you finish your task. On the other hand, don't over arch your back trying to stand tall and while bending over at the same time to reach the vacuum handle.

The best way to vacuum safely is to take a fencing stance, with one foot forward and one back. Your forward knee can be slightly bent. One hand on the vacuum handle is enough. Now use the other hand on your bent knee for added support. Keep your pelvis level and you'll do the vacuuming in record time with no pain. You can also try switching sides to even the load. For best balance always keep your right foot forward when your left hand is on the vacuum and vice versa.

If you have to vacuum under a table or furniture the best choice often is to go down on one knee with your other leg bent in a half kneel. This lets you work under the furniture without over stressing your back.

Laundry

When taking laundry out of a dryer instead of bending and rounding your back, try putting one leg out behind, leaning on the top of the dryer with one hand, and removing the dry clothes with the other. This way your back will stay fairly straight and relieve any pressure on your spine. Then when carrying the basket, be sure to pick it up from a squat and lift with your legs.

Dishes

If you wash dishes by hand at your house, try this. Before starting, open the cupboard door below the sink. As you start washing, lift one foot up and put it on the four inch raised bottom of that cupboard. This will help level your pelvis and reduce strain. You may also want to tense your buttock muscles and push your pelvis level and firmly against the counter.

Making the Bed

Making the bed is a back breaker. Never an easy or quick job it can be super-tough on backs. Be sure to avoid slumping or arching your back when you bed make. A good tip is to drop a pillow at the corner of the bed, kneel on it and smooth out the sheets and blankets while kneeling. It makes it a lot easier, you're in a good position to do the job and it's a lot less of a strain on your back.

Pregnancy and Sciatica

Pregnancy causes a lot of changes in a woman's body. One of those changes is the physical shifting of the spine to accommodate the change in the woman's center of balance and the increased "front load" of an advanced pregnancy.

To give a woman a chance to maintain her balance, the spine must accept much more weight than normal along with the related stress on the vertebrae and the associated ligaments and muscles.

Adding to this structural problem are the hormones that are being released.

One of these hormones is released during pregnancy to relax and loosen the pelvic ligaments. This is so on birth day the baby's head can move through the birth canal easier. The big problem is that this hormone, relaxin, also loosens up the sacroiliac and other joints in the same general area which can cause you more problems.

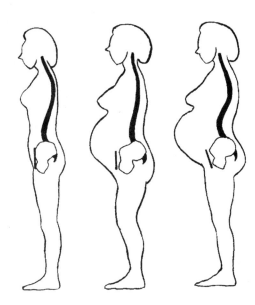

So, pregnancy does create some new problems for the spinal column. It can further irritate an already hurting sciatic nerve, or it can create a painful sciatic condition all on its own.

So, what can be done? Several things. Your best position for being comfortable while lying down during this time is most likely going to be on your side. The side position is also usually going to be the best one for sleeping or making love as well. If your sciatica is hurting and you can find one position that gives you relief from the pain and the weight of the baby, use that position. What works well for one woman might not work at all for another.

If you start experiencing back pain during pregnancy your first stop should be the obstetrician. This is just in case the back pain is caused by something other than your pregnancy or the sciatica. X-rays are prohibited during your first four or five months, depending on your doctor. If no new problems are found, stick to your exercise program and get relief from the sciatica as your doctor prescribes.

Remember, since you're pregnant the doctor won't be giving you any serious pain medication. If the pain is too great, you might ask your doctor about a special corset designed for pregnant women to help reduce back pain. Heat and massage sometimes do wonders, including that long soak in a warm tub of water. You'll be continuing your regular program of swimming, walking or biking. But as always check with your doctor first before doing any activity.

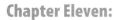

Chapter Eleven:

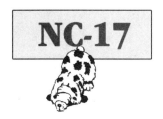

Intimacy With a Hurting Back

Having sciatica doesn't mean you have to say goodbye to your sex life. Even with a back that is prone to causing you pain you can have a satisfying and active life in the bedroom. It's time to put away the "Not tonight, honey, I've got a damn back ache again" excuse and learn how to hop back into that saddle again.

If you had a healthy sex life before your back injury, there's no reason you can't maintain it as your back gets better. There are certainly some precautions you should take, but they are nothing drastic. We'll get to those later.

If the way you usually make love causes you only a little pain and it's something you can live with, there's no reason you should change your positions or your tactics. On the other hand, if your usual positions give you so much pain you can't continue, then it's time to look for some new positions which I will go over soon.

The first step is truly believing that you can be as good a lover as you ever were. This is half the battle. Feeling unsure of yourself and anticipating pain is not going to lead to good sex.

Second, if you do need to make some changes, talk it over with your spouse. A loving partner will be ready and willing to make adjustments that will help continue your good sexual experiences. Be direct, clear and make it plain that a little adjustment now will make things better for both of you.

Third. Although there might be some days that intercourse is out of the question you CAN get creative coming up with some new ways to achieve mutually satisfying sexual experiences without the actual act of penetration. Think about it. Oral and manual stimulation can be very satisfying for both partners.

A Backache Kind of Lover

So, what's next? What will hurt and what won't?

If your lovemaking is working and not painful in spite of your hurting back or your sciatica, go right on in the same pattern. You may want to try something different just for variety even so, and the positions shown in the next couple of pages will be safe for most people with back pains. But first some precautions and tips:

- In any position, avoid an extreme swayback. This concave position can hurt your spine and if you have sciatica or other spine issues it's bound to cause you fits of pain. Keep your spine straight or only slightly bent forward during intercourse.

- Never bend forward with your knees straight, not even if you are in a lying position. This puts a great deal of force on your lumbar spinal area. It also stretches your sciatic nerve and you don't need this since it's already an issue for you. You can curve your spine forward a little, as long as your knees are bent.

- Avoid positions like lying flat on your back or on your stomach with your hips extended out straight. This includes the standard missionary position. This position will stress and stretch your psoas muscles that run from the front of your spine to just below your hip. This muscle helps control a woman's vaginal contractions.

- Whenever you can, use a position in which your hips are flexed, which will help you to avoid aggravating your lower back.

Certain positions are generally better than others for those of us that have a bad back. Following are some suggested positions. Experiment and see what works best for your and your partner.

Position 1

This is generally the best position for either partner with back pain. The partners are lying on their sides. The male is behind in a close spoon fashion. Neither has to support the weight of the other one. The woman should be careful to avoid getting into a swayback position. This position can often be used even if you have a serious backache and long-term pain.

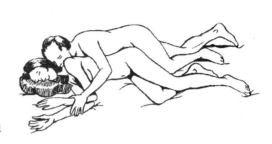

Position 2

This one is a good choice for the woman with back pain. She lies on her back with upper torso supported with pillows. The man kneels between her legs, which are bent and pulled up with her feet resting on the bed. The male supports her thighs with his thighs and his hands.

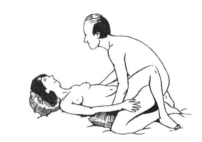

Position 3

This is another good one for the woman with a painful back. The man lies on his back with his feet spread. The woman kneels on top with her hips flexed. She must avoid getting a swayback by leaning forward and supporting her shoulders with her hands near his shoulders. The man's head and torso should be lifted with a few pillows to slightly flex his spine.

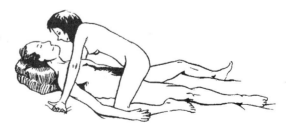

This is also a good position for the man with a hurting back.

Position 4

This one is similar to position number three. The woman kneels at his waist but faces his feet. The woman can support her body with her hands on his thighs or knees or on the bed. She should be careful not to irritate the man's back by putting too much pressure on his knees. Communicate with each other. It's important to let your partner know if you are uncomfortable or in pain at any time.

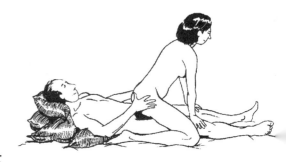

Position 5

This position is good for guys with a backache. The woman is on all fours; the man kneels behind her resting his weight on his hands or on the bed at her sides. His back should be slightly rounded.

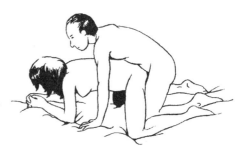

Position 6

This is another good one for the guy with a hurt back. The woman is lying on her back on the edge of the bed with both feet resting on the floor. The man kneels between her legs and supports his upper torso with his forearms on the bed beside the woman. This reduces the strain on the spine and the psoas muscle. However his is NOT a good position for the woman with back pain.

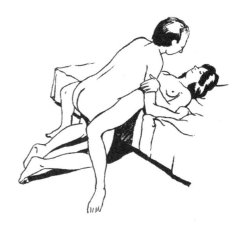

Getting Back in the Saddle Again

Many couples hold off on lovemaking when one or the other has a serious back problem. Good idea. But when the partner with back pain is on the mend, when the pain is controllable, when the urge is there and the back isn't all that bad, give sex a try.

Use the best method for the first time, probably the spoon position, Position 1. It just might work, and if so, that will be one more step in getting you back to normal.

If one of these positions doesn't work, try some of those other creative methods we talked about that can give satisfaction without actual intercourse.

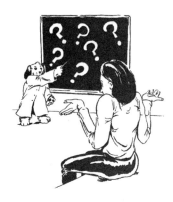

Appendix I:

Questions About Your Sciatica

If you don't ask you'll never find out. I have included here some common questions that people have about sciatica and other back problems along with some helpful answers. Maybe some of them will answer some questions you have about your own sciatica.

Be sure to keep in mind that nothing written here is designed to be a substitute for your visit to your own doctor.

Q. *If I sit all day on my thick wallet, can that have any effect on my back and my sciatica?*

A. It certainly can. By sitting on your wallet it can throw your balance off and you'll be compensating for the tilt to one side or the other. This can put a strain on your back and could even help to bring on a sciatica attack. Most pants are made so the wallet is not that far under the buttocks. The wallet can be more to the side. If your pants are not constructed that way, carry your wallet in your jacket pocket. You might also want to check out the pockets when you buy new pants.

Q. *Why is my grandmother now shorter than she was when she was a young woman?*

A. There are twenty-three discs between your vertebrae. These pillows or shock absorbers are usually somewhere around three-sixteenths of an inch thick. As a person gets older, there is a gradual wearing away and compressing of these discs. By the age of sixty, many individuals have lost as much as one-eighth of an inch from each of those pads. That means that your grandmother could be several inches shorter now at seventy years than she was when she was thirty. Some doctors refer to this as degenerative changes. Usually this doesn't cause a lot of trouble, unless the disc vanishes altogether and the vertebrae start grinding against each other.

Q. *Can large breasts contribute to back pain?*

A. Yes. Excessively large breasts can cause several problems including headaches, neck strain, low back pain, aching shoulders and even tingling in the fingers. The added weight of large breasts can shift a woman's center of gravity forward which puts a big strain on the lower back muscles and more pressure on the lower and upper back. Many times women with large breasts will try to diminish their appearance by rolling their shoulders forward and in and even rounding the spine. This can increase the pressure on the back. Many women with this condition investigate breast reduction to help solve the back and neck problems. Talk with your doctor and with a plastic surgeon to find out if this procedure will help you.

Q. *I've heard about CAT scans and a CT scan. What's the difference? Which one is best?*

A. There is no difference. CAT and CT are simply two different terms for the same thing. Most ordinary folks like us use the term CAT scan, while many doctors and nurses say CT scan. The initials stand for Computerized Axial Tomography. That simply means it's a diagnostic form of radiology. It is becoming more and more common and in back problem cases can be used to find a herniated or prolapsed disc that an X-ray can't see. The X-ray shows only bones, while the CAT scan can give a good rendering of soft tissue such as the discs between your vertebrae.

The CAT scan takes about twenty minutes to picture your spine. It is used many times in place of a myelogram and is less invasive and less painful.

Q. *My father had two herniated discs and they fused his spine. He was miserable for the last ten years of his life. Does this mean that I'll have herniated discs as well?*

A. There is no firm evidence that this is true. Many discs herniate because of the activity of the patient not from some hereditary precondition. If you do the same construction work your father did, you have a chance of getting the same problem. If he was in construction but the heaviest thing you lift is a mouse on your computer, you just might never have a ruptured disc.

Q. *I'm getting over a herniated disc. Does this mean that I might get another one soon?*

A. Yes and no. If you are working at the same job, lifting the same loads, behaving in the same way physically that you did just before you herniated the disc the first time, it well could happen again in the same disc or in another one nearby. To prevent this, take better care of your back, practice good posture, and take all the practical precautions against irritating and damaging your spinal column.

Q. *I have a backache. Should I go directly to a specialist?*

A. No. It's usually best to go to your GP or family doctor first and tell him your troubles and what hurts. This first doctor will do a preliminary examination, ask you a lot of questions and probably will have you do some exercises that can pinpoint certain back problems. If he thinks you need to see an expert on the spine, he will send you along. If your problem is minor and one that he can help you with, you'll find relief with him.

Q. *What's an osteopath? I've never heard of one.*

A. The term is better known in some states than in others. In some states the osteopath physician is on an equal footing with an M.D. They work in the same clinics and hospitals, have the same public respect, and treat the same diseases and conditions. Both can prescribe medications and do surgery. The osteopath is more likely to try non-surgical methods where possible and may not rely on medications as much as an M.D.

In some states the Osteopath can't work in M.D. hospitals. This is by state licensing practices. In those states the osteopaths have their own hospitals, agencies and organizations.

Q. *My friend says chiropractors are great healers, but some just have a bad name. Is that true?*

A. In the chiropractic field there is a wide range of skilled people. They range all the way from fine healers, to the fair, to the bad and the careless, to the out and out charlatans. Pretty much the same as any field. Many chiropractors will try to set you up with a structured program of eight, ten, twelve even twenty-four visits to take care of a problem. If you want to go to a chiropractor, check carefully into his or her qualifications, talk to patients, and know exactly what care you want from the chiropractor. As a gentle reminder, for any ailment, it's usually good to go to your family M.D. first. He or she has better training to do a complete diagnosis of any problem you may have.

Q. *If ninety percent of back problems go away in two months, why should I go to a doctor at all?*

A. True, most back pains will either go away or become much less severe in sixty days as the body works at healing itself. However, those sixty, days can be pure hell in many cases. The doctor visit will help you to deal with the pain through medications or physical therapy or other suggestions. Also, if you are one of those ten percent who has a herniated disc that must be treated, it's better to know about it right away, rather than waiting out the two months of pain, only to find out you're one of the unlucky ten percent.

Q. *I've heard of a bone scan in conjunction with sciatica. What is a bone scan? It sounds scary.*

A. A bone scan is a type of X-ray that gives you little radiation exposure. A drawback is that it takes four hours to complete. During a bone scan you'll need to lie face down on a table for a whole hour. A bone scan will show healed fractures, tumors and infections, and arthritis in the joints and bones of your spine. Routine X-rays of your low back give you ten times as much radiation exposure as a bone scan.

Q. *What's an MRI? I hear one can cost $4,000. Is this true?*

A. The letters MRI stand for Magnetic Resonance Imaging. It is not an X-ray. It uses magnetic fields and radio waves. It can give doctors pictures of the spine or other parts of the body from different angles and views. It can show plainly if a disc is herniated. It will highlight problems with the spine, tumors or other ailments and even give evidence of diseased tissue. Costs vary according to the length of time needed to do the MRI scan. Some costs can be as much as $4,000, but most are much less.

Q. *How soon can I get back to work after a bad sciatica attack?*

A. That depends on a lot of factors. Primary is what work are you doing? If you're laying eighteen-pound concrete blocks you won't be back at work for a month, maybe two. If you work in an office setting you might get back on the job two weeks after your pain is manageable. It depends on your job, your ability to work with a little pain, and how much you need that paycheck.

Q. *Is it true that an acupressurist is only an acupuncturist who uses his thumbs and fingers instead of needles on the same pressure points?*

A. Some people will say yes. Some no. Basically the two systems seem to be remarkably similar using the same body areas and pressure or needles with electrical input to establish the same overload on major nerves. How close together they are is up for speculation. Number wise there are many more practitioners with the needles than without.

Q. *If I wear high-heeled shoes, will it hurt my back?*

A. If you wear five or six inch spikes, it's going to be bad for your back as long as you're standing or walking. The heels throw the entire body out of balance and the tendency is to compensate with a swayback position causing stress on your back.

If you stick to two inch heels, there is far less chance that the swayback problem will come up. However even low heels can cause you some backache. If it doesn't, feel free to wear them but try wearing them for as short a period as possible. A spare pair of shoes at the office with lower heels or even flats is a good plan. Also a good pair of sneakers for that walk to the subway or to your parking lot is always a healthy choice.

Q. *I heard my doctor talking about the two-year sciatic rule. What is that?*

A. There is a general opinion among doctors specializing in back problems that most patients who have sciatica attacks will have another one within two years. The figure is about sixty percent. But a good percentage of that sixty percent probably didn't take care of their backs after the first attack. You bought this book and you won't make that mistake so you are more likely to find yourself in the attack free forty percent. Good back care and exercises to strengthen back muscles will take you a long way towards preventing a second sciatic attack.

Q. *Why did my doctor tell me to quit the stretching exercises I was doing? I thought it was good for my back.*

A. Probably it would be good for a well back. If you have back pain or sciatica, some stretches actually stretch the sciatic nerve and this can increase your problem and your pain.

Q. *I heard people with backaches used to use gravity boots. What ever happened to them?*

A. With gravity boots the idea is to hang upside down. This can be done a variety of ways. Some experts like the idea. Others say that it can cause a few other problems not related to stretching out your spine. Some are: increase in blood pressure and heart rate. Nerves in your ankles can show irritation and with prolonged upside down hanging, you could suffer bleeding in the back of the eye.

Q. *How much of the disc is removed in surgery?*

A. Usually only the herniated part and maybe twenty percent of the soft matter in the center of the disc. All loose material is removed. Almost never is the whole disc removed. That would leave nothing to separate the vertebrae and you'd be in bigger trouble than ever. Usually there is enough of the disc and soft core left to do the shock absorbing job the disc was designed to do.

Q. *My friend with sciatica said he didn't try to have sex for six months after his back felt better. Isn't that too long to wait?*

A. Sexual intercourse can and should be undertaken as soon as the person feels ready. If the sciatic pain is mostly gone, try the spoon position described in a previous chapter. Be careful not to bend your back, always bend your hips. If your first attempt causes too much pain, wait a while. Six months is way too long.

Q. *I'm having a discotomy. Can I give my blood for use during my surgery?*

A. Almost always. Most hospitals will draw your blood before surgery and hold it for use when you go in the operating room. Check with your hospital for their time frames and schedules and about costs. Most people feel more secure using their own blood if any is required during surgery. Find out how many pints are usually needed and plan ahead.

Q. *I like to sleep on my stomach, but my wife says that's hard on my back. Is she right?*

A. If you use pillows in the right places, you can still sleep on your stomach. Use a pillow for your head that will keep your head in a straight line with your back, not pushed up or dropped down. Then support your stomach with a pillow or a lumbar roll. Fasten this around your waist so it will support your stomach or your back if you turn over during the night.

Q. *Why is it better to push a heavy object than to pull it?*

A. When you push a couch or a big box, you can dig in your feet and use your body weight as well as the thrust of your muscles to push an item. On the other hand when you try to pull something, you have only your muscles to do the job. You're short half of your resources. So always push, instead of pull.

Q. *Is hypnosis pure quackery or is there some value?*

A. Many people use hypnosis to alter their state of mind with the hope that this will help alter their physical side. For some, it works, for others it is not quite right. Learn as much as you can about hypnotism, then go to a registered hypnotist and have that person hypnotize you. Get the feel of it. If you like it, get training so you can hypnotize yourself. Hypnotism might not cure your sciatic back, but for some people it can help them to endure the pain and to take a different approach to it.

Q. *After an injury or pain, is it ice first or heat first?*

A. Watch pro football. The ice pack comes on the moment an injured player hits the sidelines. Ice tends to reduce swelling and to downgrade pain. The use of heat comes a day later to bring fresh blood to the injured area to speed the recovery. After the first day some people think that alternating heat and ice packs helps speed recovery.

Q. *Whatever happened to that month long bed rest plan after a sciatica attack?*

A. It went out with the polyester suit. Times change, we learn. The long-term bed rest was finally determined to cause more problems than the good it did. The back is a functional mechanism. It isn't functioning when lying in bed. Normal use of the spine, after a day or two of bed rest, turned out to be the best for the patient. Problems such as bedsores, a deterioration of muscles for walking and sitting up all led to the cutting bed rest from thirty days to two by most doctors.

Q. *I saw a headline about a $300 injection that can do the job of a $10,000 back surgery. What does that mean?*

A. That is chymopapain, a substance that is injected into the disc that "melts down" the soft core of the disc that has prolapsed or herniated and is pressing against the sciatic nerve root causing the pain. When the material there melts from the shot, it is carried away by the blood and eventually discharged from the body in urine. This does the same thing a discotomy does, except it is done simply, is less intrusive, creates no blood loss or healing of surgical procedures, and costs only about $300. A discotomy with doctors and operating room and all usually costs about $10,000. Many doctors are now looking at the injection as a good substitute for the discotomy. It is much easier on the patient, from a pain and suffering, recovery and a financial basis.

Q. *Does a bulging disc always mean the person has back pain?*

A. No. Recent studies show that with MRI and CAT Scan, many patients are found to have herniated discs and bulging discs, yet they have no back pain. In persons over forty, it was found that fifty percent of them had bulging discs but no pain. In another study thirty five percent of persons checked who were over forty had herniated discs yet no pain. Here the spinal canal was probably large enough to allow for the herniation or bulging so it did not press hard on the root nerve to cause any pain.

Q. *With all this talk about the back and the spine, isn't it a rather delicate structure we should treat with care?*

A. Not at all. Actually the spine is a finely built foundation for the back that can take a lot of pressure, and withstand tremendous forces without injury. The secret is to be sure that the muscles that support the back are kept strong with good flexibility and endurance. These are maintained with the correct body mechanics and good posture.

Q. *Is it true that it puts more strain on your back to sit than it does to stand? How can that be?*

A. Yes, true. Standing is easier on your back. It's the mechanics of the thing. By sitting there is more weight concentrated on the lower back than when standing. It's a matter of weight and muscle use and tension and all that sort of scientific stuff. Sitting is harder on a back, especially if it's an already hurting back.

Q. *I've heard that the older a person gets, the worse the back becomes and more pain and misery. Is this right?*

A. You heard it wrong. The fact is that back pain and problems peak in the thirty-five to fifty-five years of your life. After that back pain and problems actually decrease for most people. Now the spine will continue to degenerate as the discs shrink and wear away. That's why older people get shorter. But as far as backs and the spine problems getting worse and worse in the sixties, seventies and eighties, it just isn't so.

Q. *A friend told me that because of my back pain, I should go to his doctor because he started out with an X-ray of the spine and back to be sure everything was right. Is this the usual procedure?*

A. No. Most doctors go through their regular diagnosis procedure for patients with back pain to try to tie down the cause and the problem. This usually is after two or three weeks of conservative treatment of two days of rest, then medications, and other conservative methods. If these do not solve the problem or show the cause, then the X-ray is usually used. These days the X-ray might not be used and a CAT scan given instead since it's a better diagnostic tool in many ways.

Q. *Why would a doctor use psychological testing when working on a diagnosis for back pain? Seems weird.*

A. Some doctors find a need for psychological testing if the patient does not respond to other methods. Psychological testing can be used for several reasons. Among them: if the patient has serious depression or anxiety, if there is substance abuse such as alcohol, drugs or addiction to prescription drugs, lack of the ability to cope with pain, or it's suspected the pain may be partly stress related. Not weird at all.

Q. *What good is ultrasound in back treatment?*

A. Ultrasound does much the same thing as moist heat. It warms the tissue and simply reduces some pain and makes you feel better. Ultrasound is the use of sound waves with a higher frequency than the human ear can hear. The ultrasound waves used here are absorbed by the tissue warming it and reducing the pain. This is not a treatment to cure the problem. When ultrasound is used it is to provide short-term relief from the pain, similar to that offered by moist heat.

Q. *What is chronic opioid therapy as used for back pain?*

A. It's a controversial treatment not much used in the United States. Simply put it's the long-term use of highly addictive drugs such as opiates and morphine to control a patient's pain. Most doctors won't even consider such drastic medication because of the high incidence of addiction as well as the side effects and the patient's tolerance for the drugs. Side effects include serious constipation, insomnia, decreased sexual function, trouble thinking and focusing.

Q. *Is the antidepressant Prozac used much for back pain?*

A. Sometimes. Prozac is one of six or eight antidepressants that some doctors feel has some beneficial effect in some patients when they have depression combined with back pain. One of the reasons to use an antidepressant would be when a back patient has serious problems sleeping. Some of the antidepressant drugs will help normalize sleeping and also help reduce the pain associated with the back problems. The use of drugs such as Prozac would be in extreme cases only and for a limited time.

Q. *Is it true that sitting too long on a toilet seat can irritate an already screaming sciatic nerve?*

A. Absolutely true. Also too much straining to have a bowel movement can do the same thing. If you have or are getting over a sciatic attack here are some other ways you can strain and irritate that already hurting sciatic nerve: Don't sit on cold concrete for any length of time. Don't over-stretch before exercising, take it easy. Low, under slung car seats can irritate your sciatic nerve. Too little flesh on your bottom can irritate the sciatic nerves so if you do a lot of sitting try a good soft pillow. Even a lumpy, uneven pillow can irritate your already sensitive sciatic nerve.

Q. *Is it just an old wives' tale that hot baths will help a hurting back and sciatic problems?*

A. Not at all. A good warm bath for twenty minutes will do wonders for that hurting back. Why? The warm infusion in the body reduces stiffness in the muscles and joints and brings a rush of new blood through the affected areas. The warmth opens the blood vessels more than usual so more blood gets to muscles and into the tissue.

For another aid, try, putting a double handful of Epsom salts into your warm bath. This is magnesium sulfate and it opens your pores and induces perspiration. This helps cleans your body inside.

After twenty minutes let the Epsom salts water out and rinse off with fresh cool water from the tap. This will close up your pores and get your circulation back in balance. Then get out of the tub slowly. You may feel a little lightheaded and you don't want to risk passing out.

Q. *My purse gets heavy sometimes. Can this hurt my sore back?*

A. You bet it can hurt. Dump out your purse and leave at home everything you don't absolutely need to take with you. Try using one of your smaller purses so you can't overload it. Be sure to shift even a shoulder strap purse from side to side during the day. If you have lots to carry, do it with a backpack instead of a briefcase. Might not be as fashionable, but it's much easier on your back, and they might think you're still in school.

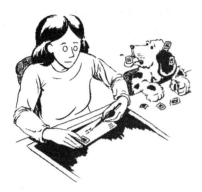

Appendix II:

Information Sources for Back Pain

There is a wealth of information available these days on almost any topic you care to research—including sciatica and back pain. Give these sources a whirl to get specific answers to questions and for general information on the spine, sciatica and back problems. For those of you on the Internet, don't forget that there are hundreds of sources you can tap for free information about backs and sciatica and all sorts of subjects. Surf the net and see.

#1. Your Family Doctor:

Phone your family doctor or your doctor in an HMO. Chances are that his office will have some literature on the back and sciatica. Tell them you're a patient and working with the doctor on your back pain and ask if they have any printed material. Most Docs will be more than happy to mail you some information.

#2. Your HMO, Health Maintenance Organization:

If you are a member of a large HMO your local HMO hospital probably has a library. Call them and ask them what they have on sciatica and back problems. They may be able to mail you material or invite you in to read their reference material in the library. Many of these are quite helpful.

#3. The U.S. Government:

National Health Information Center (NHIC) is a U.S. government service that the federal government operates that will give you information on any health problem. It may be in the form of literature or they may give you referrals to libraries or organizations. You can print materials, or order them, directly from their website as well.

Phone: (301) 565-4167 or toll free (800) 336-4797

Website: www.health.gov/nhic/

#4. International College of Acupuncture & Electrotherapeutics:

This is a nonprofit educational organization that is chartered by the University of the State of New York. It promotes research and teaching of safe and effective acupuncture and related treatments including herbal medicine. It works to combine the best of Western and Oriental medicine through international cooperation and shares its findings with the public.

Address: 800 Riverside Drive, Suite 8-1, New York, N.Y. 10032

Phone: (212) 781-6262

Fax: (212) 923-2279

#5. The American College for Advancement in Medicine (ACAM):

This not-for-profit organization educates physicians and other health care professionals on preventative and nutritional medicine. ACAM provides referrals to naturopathic physicians on its website.

Address: 23121 Verdugo Drive, Suite 204, Laguna Hills, CA 92653

Phone: (949) 583-7666 or toll-free (800) 532-3688

Website: www.acam.org

#6. American Association for Naturopathic Physicians (AANP):

This national professional society represents naturopathic physicians who are licensed (Or are eligible for licensing) as primary-care providers. Referrals to a naturopath in your area are available through it's website. Naturopaths are trained as specialists in the use of natural therapeutics and restoring overall health. Where required, they must pass a state licensing examination. Naturopathic medicine blends centuries-old therapies with current advances in the study of health, concentrating on whole-patient wellness.

Address: 3201 New Mexico Avenue, N.W. Suite 350, Washington, DC 20016

Phone: (202) 895-1392 or toll-free (866) 538-2267

E-mail: member.services@naturopathic.org

Website: www.naturopathic.org

#7. Health World Online:

Offers vast resources in nutrition, fitness, self-care and mind/body approaches to maintaining high-level health.

Address: 171 Pier Ave., #160, Santa Monica, CA 90405

Email: info@healthy.net

Website: www.healthy.net

#8. Journal of Alternative and Complementary Medicine:

The journal includes observational and analytical reports on treatments outside the realm of allopathic medicine, which are gaining interest and warranting research to assess their therapeutic value. This organization publishes a monthly newsletter devoted to alternative and complementary medicine.

Address: 2 Madison Ave., Larchmont, NY 10538

Phone: (914) 834-3100

Fax: (914) 834-3688

Website: www.liebertpub.com

#9. National Association for Holistic Aromatherapy:

Publishes a quarterly "Aroma-therapy Journal."

Address: 3327 W. Indian Trail Road PMB 144, Spokane, WA 99208

Phone: (509) 325-3419

Fax: (509) 325-3479

Email: info@naha.org

Website: www.naha.org

#10. Association for Applied Psychophysiology & Biofeedback (AAPB):

The AAPB pursues continuing study in biofeedback. It has over two thousand members around the U.S. It can provide referrals for you to locate qualified professionals in your area.

Address: 10200 West 44th Ave., Suite 304, Wheat Ridge, CO 80033-2840

Phone: (303) 422-8436 or toll free (800) 477-8892

Fax: (303) 422-8894

Email: aapb@resourcecenter.com

Website: www.aapb.org

#11. American Botanical Council:

The Council conducts research and education supporting herbal folk remedies, teas and other herb based products. It also publishes a quarterly newsletter.

Address: 6200 Manor Road, Austin, TX 78723

Phone: (512) 926-4900

Fax: (512) 926-2345

Email: abc@herbalgram.org

Website: www.herbalgram.org

#12. American Herbal Products Association (AHPA):

The AHPA promotes the responsible commerce of products that contain herbs. Their Botanical Safety Handbook contains safety data for more than 600 commonly sold herbs.

Address: 8484 Georgia Ave., Suite 370, Silver Spring, MD 20910

Phone: (301) 588-1171

Fax: (301) 588-1174

Email: ahpa@ahpa.org

Website: www.ahpa.org

#13. National Center for Homeopathy:

A non-profit membership organization dedicated to making homeopathy accessible to the public. Their mission is to promote health through homeopathy. Their magazine "Homeopathy Today" contains up-to-date news, tips, short articles and a calendar of events. Their library is one of the largest collections of homeopathic literature in the United States.

Address: 801 N Fairfax St., Suite 306, Alexandria, VA 22314

Phone: (703) 548-7790

Fax: (703) 548-7792

Email: info@homeopathic.org

Website: www.homeopathic.org

#14. Certification Board for Nutrition Specialists (CBNS):

The CBNS helps establish standards and certifies nutritionists who are able to pass an examination. The board can provide a list of qualified professional nutritionists in your area.

Address: 300 S. Duncan Ave., Suite 225, Clearwater, FL 33755

Phone: (727) 446-6086

Fax: (727) 446-6202

Email: office@cert-nutrition.org

Website: www.cbns.org

#15. National Institute of Mental Health (NIMH):

This federal agency is a great resource for information on stress control and any behavioral disorders.

Address: National Institute of Mental Health (NIMH), Public Information and Communications Branch, 6001 Executive Boulevard, Room 8184, MSC 9663, Bethesda, MD 20892-9663

Phone: (301) 443-4513

Fax: (301) 443-8431

Email: nimhinfo@nih.gov

Website: www.nimh.nih.gov

#16. The National Council on Alcoholism and Drug Dependence (NCADD):

For help with any kind of alcohol or drug addiction, aid, referrals, local organizations, information, literature, prevention, intervention and treatment.

Address: 22 Cortlandt Street, Suite 801, New York, NY 10007-3128

Phone: (212) 269-7797

Fax: (212)-269-7510

Hope Line: (800) NCA-CALL (24-hour referral)

Email: national@ncadd.org

Website: www.ncadd.org

#17. More general information about sciatica is obtainable from the following sciatica websites. You also can simply type SCIATICA into your browser:

www.sciatica.org

www.nlm.nih.gov/medlineplus/sciatica.html

www.mayoclinic.com/health/sciatica/DS00516

en.wikipedia.org/wiki/Sciatica

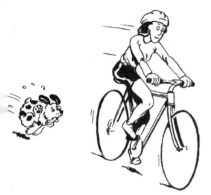

Appendix III:

Exercise and Aerobic Charts for Your Recordkeeping

O n the following pages you'll find charts, one for every day of the next year, so you can chart out your daily exercise and/or aerobic activity. The key at the bottom shows your level of work. They go from level 1 through 10 showing how many repetitions you do on each one. Enjoy.

AEROBICS

Type	Time	Weight

EXERCISE #   LEVEL___

Date	Warm	1	2	3	4	5	6	7	8	9	10	11	12	13	14	15	16	17	18	19	20	21	22	23	24	Cool
1																										
2																										
3																										
4																										
5																										
6																										
7																										
8																										
9																										
10																										
11																										
12																										
13																										
14																										
15																										
16																										
17																										
18																										
19																										
20																										
21																										
22																										
23																										
24																										
25																										
26																										
27																										
28																										
29																										
30																										

AEROBICS

EXERCISE # **LEVEL____**

Date	Warm	1	2	3	4	5	6	7	8	9	10	11	12	13	14	15	16	17	18	19	20	21	22	23	24	Cool	Type	Time	Weight
1																														
2																														
3																														
4																														
5																														
6																														
7																														
8																														
9																														
10																														
11																														
12																														
13																														
14																														
15																														
16																														
17																														
18																														
19																														
20																														
21																														
22																														
23																														
24																														
25																														
26																														
27																														
28																														
29																														
30																														
31																														

Development Levels: #1-4 reps, #2-6 reps, #3-8 reps, #4-10 reps, #5-12 reps, #6-16 reps, #7-18 reps, #8-20 reps, #9-22 reps, #10-24 reps

		AEROBICS		
		Type	Time	Weight

	EXERCISE # LEVEL___																							
Date	Warm	1	2	3	4	5	6	7	8	9	10	11	12	13	14	15	16	17	18	19	20	21	22	23	24	Cool
1																										
2																										
3																										
4																										
5																										
6																										
7																										
8																										
9																										
10																										
11																										
12																										
13																										
14																										
15																										
16																										
17																										
18																										
19																										
20																										
21																										
22																										
23																										
24																										
25																										
26																										
27																										
28																										
29																										
30																										

EXERCISE # LEVEL___ | AEROBICS

Date	Warm	1	2	3	4	5	6	7	8	9	10	11	12	13	14	15	16	17	18	19	20	21	22	23	24	Cool	Type	Time	Weight
1																													
2																													
3																													
4																													
5																													
6																													
7																													
8																													
9																													
10																													
11																													
12																													
13																													
14																													
15																													
16																													
17																													
18																													
19																													
20																													
21																													
22																													
23																													
24																													
25																													
26																													
27																													
28																													
29																													
30																													
31																													

Development Levels: #1-4 reps, #2-6 reps, #3-8 reps, #4-10 reps, #5-12 reps, #6-16 reps, #7-18 reps, #8-20 reps, #9-22 reps, #10-24 reps

		AEROBICS		
		Type	Time	Weight

EXERCISE # LEVEL____																									AEROBICS		
Date	Warm	1	2	3	4	5	6	7	8	9	10	11	12	13	14	15	16	17	18	19	20	21	22	23	24	Cool	Type	Time	Weight
1																													
2																													
3																													
4																													
5																													
6																													
7																													
8																													
9																													
10																													
11																													
12																													
13																													
14																													
15																													
16																													
17																													
18																													
19																													
20																													
21																													
22																													
23																													
24																													
25																													
26																													
27																													
28																													
29																													
30																													

EXERCISE # _____ LEVEL _____ **AEROBICS**

Date	Warm	1	2	3	4	5	6	7	8	9	10	11	12	13	14	15	16	17	18	19	20	21	22	23	24	Cool	Type	Time	Weight
1																													
2																													
3																													
4																													
5																													
6																													
7																													
8																													
9																													
10																													
11																													
12																													
13																													
14																													
15																													
16																													
17																													
18																													
19																													
20																													
21																													
22																													
23																													
24																													
25																													
26																													
27																													
28																													
29																													
30																													
31																													

Development Levels: #1-4 reps, #2-6 reps, #3-8 reps, #4-10 reps, #5-12 reps, #6-16 reps, #7-18 reps, #8-20 reps, #9-22 reps, #10-24 reps

EXERCISE # LEVEL____ | AEROBICS

Date	Warm	1	2	3	4	5	6	7	8	9	10	11	12	13	14	15	16	17	18	19	20	21	22	23	24	Cool	Type	Time	Weight
1																													
2																													
3																													
4																													
5																													
6																													
7																													
8																													
9																													
10																													
11																													
12																													
13																													
14																													
15																													
16																													
17																													
18																													
19																													
20																													
21																													
22																													
23																													
24																													
25																													
26																													
27																													
28																													
29																													
30																													

EXERCISE # _____   LEVEL _____

AEROBICS

Date	Warm	1	2	3	4	5	6	7	8	9	10	11	12	13	14	15	16	17	18	19	20	21	22	23	24	Cool	Type	Time	Weight
1																													
2																													
3																													
4																													
5																													
6																													
7																													
8																													
9																													
10																													
11																													
12																													
13																													
14																													
15																													
16																													
17																													
18																													
19																													
20																													
21																													
22																													
23																													
24																													
25																													
26																													
27																													
28																													
29																													
30																													
31																													

Development Levels: #1-4 reps, #2-6 reps, #3-8 reps, #4-10 reps, #5-12 reps, #6-16 reps, #7-18 reps, #8-20 reps, #9-22 reps, #10-24 reps

		AEROBICS		
		Type	Time	Weight

EXERCISE # LEVEL ___																									
Date	Warm	1	2	3	4	5	6	7	8	9	10	11	12	13	14	15	16	17	18	19	20	21	22	23	24	Cool
1																									
2																									
3																									
4																									
5																									
6																									
7																									
8																									
9																									
10																									
11																									
12																									
13																									
14																									
15																									
16																									
17																									
18																									
19																									
20																									
21																									
22																									
23																									
24																									
25																									
26																									
27																									
28																									
29																									
30																									

EXERCISE #   LEVEL___   AEROBICS

Date	Warm	1	2	3	4	5	6	7	8	9	10	11	12	13	14	15	16	17	18	19	20	21	22	23	24	Cool	Type	Time	Weight
1																													
2																													
3																													
4																													
5																													
6																													
7																													
8																													
9																													
10																													
11																													
12																													
13																													
14																													
15																													
16																													
17																													
18																													
19																													
20																													
21																													
22																													
23																													
24																													
25																													
26																													
27																													
28																													
29																													
30																													
31																													

Development Levels: #1-4 reps, #2-6 reps, #3-8 reps, #4-10 reps, #5-12 reps, #6-16 reps, #7-18 reps, #8-20 reps, #9-22 reps, #10-24 reps

AEROBICS

Weight	Time	Type

EXERCISE #   LEVEL____

Date	Warm	1	2	3	4	5	6	7	8	9	10	11	12	13	14	15	16	17	18	19	20	21	22	23	24	Cool
1																										
2																										
3																										
4																										
5																										
6																										
7																										
8																										
9																										
10																										
11																										
12																										
13																										
14																										
15																										
16																										
17																										
18																										
19																										
20																										
21																										
22																										
23																										
24																										
25																										
26																										
27																										
28																										
29																										
30																										

AEROBICS

EXERCISE # ___ LEVEL ___

Date	Warm	1	2	3	4	5	6	7	8	9	10	11	12	13	14	15	16	17	18	19	20	21	22	23	24	Cool	Type	Time	Weight
1																													
2																													
3																													
4																													
5																													
6																													
7																													
8																													
9																													
10																													
11																													
12																													
13																													
14																													
15																													
16																													
17																													
18																													
19																													
20																													
21																													
22																													
23																													
24																													
25																													
26																													
27																													
28																													
29																													
30																													
31																													

Development Levels: #1–4 reps, #2–6 reps, #3–8 reps, #4–10 reps, #5–12 reps, #6–16 reps, #7–18 reps, #8–20 reps, #9–22 reps, #10–24 reps

Date	Warm	1	2	3	4	5	6	7	8	9	10	11	12	13	14	15	16	17	18	19	20	21	22	23	24	Cool	Type	Time	Weight
1																														
2																														
3																														
4																														
5																														
6																														
7																														
8																														
9																														
10																														
11																														
12																														
13																														
14																														
15																														
16																														
17																														
18																														
19																														
20																														
21																														
22																														
23																														
24																														
25																														
26																														
27																														
28																														
29																														
30																														

EXERCISE #   LEVEL____

AEROBICS

EXERCISE #   LEVEL ___   AEROBICS

Date	Warm	1	2	3	4	5	6	7	8	9	10	11	12	13	14	15	16	17	18	19	20	21	22	23	24	Cool	Type	Time	Weight
1																													
2																													
3																													
4																													
5																													
6																													
7																													
8																													
9																													
10																													
11																													
12																													
13																													
14																													
15																													
16																													
17																													
18																													
19																													
20																													
21																													
22																													
23																													
24																													
25																													
26																													
27																													
28																													
29																													
30																													
31																													

Development Levels: #1–4 reps, #2–6 reps, #3-8 reps, #4-10 reps, #5-12 reps, #6-16 reps, #7–18 reps, #8-20 reps, #9-22 reps, #10-24 reps

				EXERCISE #							LEVEL____																	AEROBICS			
Date	Warm	1	2	3	4	5	6	7	8	9	10	11	12	13	14	15	16	17	18	19	20	21	22	23	24	Cool	Type	Time	Weight
1																													
2																													
3																													
4																													
5																													
6																													
7																													
8																													
9																													
10																													
11																													
12																													
13																													
14																													
15																													
16																													
17																													
18																													
19																													
20																													
21																													
22																													
23																													
24																													
25																													
26																													
27																													
28																													
29																													
30																													

Index

A

AAPB 146
Abdominal muscles 23, 45, 80, 81, 87, 91
Abdominals 84-86, 89, 91
ACAM 27, 144
Acupoints 31
Acupressure 36-38, 69
Acupuncture 29, 33-36, 38, 69, 144
Addiction 20, 21, 140
Advil 20, 65, 66
AHPA 146
Aleve 20, 65, 66
Alignment 98, 99, 101
  bad spine 82
  spine 42
Ankylosing Spondylitis 7
Antidepressants 140
Anti-inflammatory 55, 66
Arthritis 6, 44, 79, 133
  degenerative 6, 7
  rheumatoid 6, 7
Aspirin 66, 67

B

Backaches 105, 125, 126, 131, 134, 135
Backbone 13, 14
Balance 31, 85, 86, 88, 89, 118, 120, 129,
  134, 141
Bath, warm 33, 141
Bed 15, 22, 55, 69, 78, 113-115, 120, 125,
  126, 137
  rest 22, 66, 68, 137
Bend 12-15, 65, 81, 82, 85, 89, 90, 92, 101-
  103, 114, 119, 136
Bending tips 95-104
Bicycling 72, 73, 79
Biking 72, 121
Biofeedback 32, 69, 146
Bone scan 133
Bones 10, 11, 13-16, 22, 53, 55, 56, 60, 62,
  63, 72, 131, 133
Braces 23, 24, 62
Brain 14, 16, 32, 34, 35, 70, 115
Breasts, large 130
Breathing techniques 44, 45
Bulging discs 4-6, 9, 60, 138
Burn 70, 72, 84
Buttocks 1, 3, 5, 8, 9, 38, 62, 78, 80, 81, 86,
  87, 100, 129

C

Calories 70-73
Cancer 11, 12, 19, 23, 44
CAT scan 11, 12, 59, 63, 130, 131, 139
Chair 16, 92, 95-99, 103, 105, 106, 108
Chest 15, 69, 83, 90-92, 100, 101, 108, 117
Chinese Massage 30, 31
Chiropractic 40-44, 68, 132
Chores 111-122
Chymopapain injections 62, 63
Codeine 20
Cold packs 25, 26, 67
Computer 11, 12, 32, 96, 105, 107, 108,
  131
Control pain 47
Core muscles 45, 77

Corset 23
Country doctor 50
CT scan 8, 130
Cushions 2, 3, 6, 15, 16, 92, 116

D
Depression 3, 22, 140
Desk 47, 86, 95, 96, 99, 106, 108
Devil's Claw 54
Diagnosis 9, 11, 43, 66, 139
Diet 53-56
Digestive problems 55
Discotomy 59-61, 63, 64, 136, 138
Discs 1-7, 10-12, 15, 16, 20, 22, 23, 46, 51,
    52, 60, 63, 66, 130, 131, 133, 135, 137,
    138
Discs Bulge 2
Discs
  damaged 47
  herniate 131
  shrink 6, 139
Drugs 20, 48-51, 62, 64, 140, 141

E
Endorphins 32, 35, 39
Exercise 22, 77-94, 149-152
Exercises, abdominal 87, 91

F
Facet joints 7, 14, 61
Fat 70, 71
Flexibility 22, 46, 71, 72, 138
Fractures 11, 12
Fusion surgery 61
G
Gardening 116, 117
Good posture 86, 88, 95, 97-100, 131, 138

H
Headaches 12, 67, 97, 130
Heat 25, 26, 67, 121, 137
Herbal products 33, 146, 147
Herniated discs 3, 6, 9-12, 59, 62, 63, 66,
    131, 133, 138
Homeopathy 48-50, 70, 147

Hormones 120, 121
Hydrotherapy 32, 33
Hypnosis 46-48, 69, 137

I
Ibuprofens 20, 66, 67
Incision 60-63
Inflammation 7, 32, 39, 42, 53, 55, 68
Information sources 143-148
Injections 12, 25, 53, 63, 64, 137, 138
Intimacy 123-128

J
Job 101
Joints 6, 7, 79, 121, 133, 141
Journal 73, 145

K
Keyboard 95, 106, 107

L
Labels 70, 71
Laundry 120
Legs 10, 22, 38, 40, 51, 65, 69, 71, 80, 96,
    100, 106, 114, 117, 126
Lifting 3, 12, 68, 116, 119, 131
Ligaments 2, 22, 52, 60
Limber 89, 90
Lumbar 5, 8, 10, 17, 23, 70, 84, 99
  roll 116, 136
  vertebrae 11, 15, 17
M
Manipulation 31, 40-44, 51, 53
Massage, therapeutic 29, 30, 39, 121
Mattress 114
Medical doctors 4, 23, 29, 30, 33, 36, 41-
    44, 147, 148
Medications 3, 12, 20, 21, 27-29, 34, 36,
    48, 49, 132, 133, 139, 140, 144
  homeopathic 48-50
Medicine, complementary 145
Meditation 44, 45
Menstrual sciatic pain 8
Microdiscotomy 60, 62
Minerals 53, 54, 56

Motrin   20, 65, 66
Mowing   118
MRI   12, 59, 133, 138
Muscle
  atrophy   22
  relaxants   20, 54, 55
  spasms   6, 8
  tension   26, 32
Muscles   1, 8, 15, 17, 20, 30, 32, 52, 53, 60,
  71, 72, 77-81, 86-89, 96, 135-138, 141
  extensor   87
  gluteal   78
  hamstring   80
  psoas   126
  relaxed   32
  shortened   80
  spasming   30
  strengthen   85
  tightened   96
Musculoskeletal system   50, 52
Myelogram   12, 52, 53, 63, 131

N
Narrowing spinal canal   7, 8
National Institute of Mental Health   148
Naturopathy   27, 144, 145
Neck   3, 9, 14, 31, 82, 87, 88, 96-101, 106,
  107, 115, 117, 118
  pain   97
Nerve roots   1, 3-5, 10, 17, 53, 59, 60, 138
Nerves   3-5, 14, 16, 17, 34, 39, 56, 59, 60,
  69, 134, 135
NIMH   148
Non-traditional methods   27-58
Nucleus   62, 63
Numbness   1, 3, 8

O
Orthopaedic physicians   52, 53
Osteoarthritis   6, 7
Osteopathy   50-52, 132

P
Packs, hot   25, 26, 68
Pain   3-11, 19-21, 23-25, 29-39, 41-48, 51-
  55, 59-62, 65, 67-70, 72-74, 79, 80, 83, 84,
  123-127, 133-141, 143-148
  chronic   20, 22, 41, 59, 125
  medications   19, 35, 121
  perception of   26, 39
  relief   25, 26, 30-32, 35, 37, 47, 48, 55, 67,
    69, 70
    tips   12, 16, 22, 26, 32, 40, 45, 47, 51,
    55, 56, 62, 67, 69, 73, 75
  stress loop   73
Painkillers, natural   32, 34, 35
Painting   117, 118
Pelvis   8, 39, 62, 85-88, 96-99, 101, 120
Physical therapists   23, 25, 29
Piriformis muscle   8
Placebo effect   27-29
Planting   116, 117
Position   5, 16, 31, 68, 80, 81, 84-88, 90-92,
  96-98, 100, 115, 119-121, 123-127
  back-stressing   97
  best   99, 115, 121, 125
  change   116
  sitting   82, 84, 96, 97
  spoon   127, 136
  stressful   96, 97
  suggested   125
  swayback   118, 125, 134
Posture(s)   5, 30, 32, 44-46
Postures
  bad   95
  sitting   97, 98
Pregnancy   120, 121
Pressure   2-4, 15, 16, 23, 30, 32, 39, 51, 59,
  60, 62, 69, 82, 92, 100, 117, 130
  points   36-38, 134
Protrusion   3-5
Prozac   140, 141
Purses   142
Push   136

R
Radiation   11, 12, 133
Radiologists   11, 63
Raking leaves   117
Recovery   64, 66, 78, 137, 138

Reflexology 38-40, 69
Relief 24, 25, 29, 35, 38, 63, 66, 121, 132
Rupture 2, 3
Ruptured disc 10, 12, 20, 51, 131

S
Sciatic
   nerve 1, 4, 8, 10, 17, 32, 62, 80, 81, 135, 141
   pain 1, 2, 4, 5, 17, 51, 52, 56, 63, 81, 136
Sciatica
   attack 80, 83, 84, 105, 129, 135, 137
   pain 2, 3, 5-9, 11, 16, 17, 35, 36, 38, 46, 50, 64, 67, 69, 70, 75, 105
Self help therapy 65-76
Sensory fibers, large 25, 26
Sex 123, 127, 136
Shock absorbers 15, 16, 130
Shoulders 7, 14, 17, 31, 45, 82-86, 90, 96, 106, 108, 125, 130
Sitting and standing 95-104
Sit-ups 84
Sleep 22, 31, 46, 54, 55, 73, 111-122, 136
Snow, shoveling 118, 119
Spasm 10, 30
Spinal
   canal 4-7, 14, 36, 53, 138
   column 1, 7, 15, 16, 40, 121, 131
   cord 9, 10, 13, 14, 17, 32
   stenosis 6, 7
Spine 2, 3, 6-8, 10-18, 36, 39, 40, 45, 62, 63, 78-80, 82, 83, 87-90, 96-101, 114-116, 120, 130-133, 137-139
Spondylolisthesis 6, 7, 59, 61
Standing 6, 78, 82, 85, 86, 95-97, 99-101, 103, 117, 119, 134, 139
Strengthen 7, 31, 69, 71, 80, 86-88, 135
Stress levels 73-75
Stretch 80-83, 91, 92, 118, 135
Stretching 15, 50, 80, 82, 89, 97, 135
Supplements 53
Surgeon, orthopaedic 52, 53, 63
Surgery 23, 24, 51, 52, 59-64, 132, 135-137
   decompression 60, 61

T
TCM 30, 31
Tendons 52
Tension 26, 30, 32, 39, 83, 101, 106, 139
Therapy, chronic opioid 21, 140
Tingling 1, 8, 9, 130
Tissue
   scar 25, 61, 63
   soft 10, 52, 131
Traction 24, 53
Traditional medicine approach 19-26
Tranquilizer 54, 55
Travel 111-122
Treatments 23-25, 27, 29, 34-36, 38-40, 42, 44, 53, 60, 62, 140, 144, 145, 148
Tumors 6, 23, 59, 133
Tylenol-2 20

U
Ultrasound 25, 140

V
Vacuuming 119
Vegetables 56
Vertebrae 7, 13-15, 59-61
Vitamins 20, 53, 54, 56

W
Wallet 20, 62, 129
Water exercise 79
Wear 2, 3, 6, 60, 61, 134, 139
Weight 3, 14, 40, 45, 70-72, 84, 85, 88, 101, 105, 120, 121, 125, 126, 130, 139
Willow bark, white 55
Work
   chair 105, 106
   habits 3, 95, 105
Workout 70-72, 78, 80, 86, 91
Workplace 105-110

X
X-rays 8, 10-12, 41, 51, 52, 60, 61, 121, 131, 133, 139

Y
Yoga 44-46, 69